eat YOURSELF
young

*Take years off your looks with
this revolutionary new eating plan*

ELIZABETH
PEYTON-JONES

Editorial Director Anne Furniss
Creative Director Helen Lewis
Editor Emma Callery
Designer Katherine Case
Illustrator Katherine Case
Production Director Vincent Smith
Production Controller James Finan

First published in 2011 by
Quadrille Publishing Limited
Alhambra House, 27–31 Charing Cross Road, London WC2H 0LS
www.quadrille.co.uk

Cataloguing in Publication Data: a catalogue record for this book is available from
the British Library.

ISBN 978 184400 989 3

Printed in China

If you suffer from diabetes, heart disease, cancer or other medical conditions,
are pregnant/breastfeeding, on medication, or have difficulty metabolizing iron,
check with your GP before embarking on the EYY Eating Plan. If you suffer from
blood sugar disorders, you may need to eat more regularly than three times a day.
If you play sport intensively or are undergoing a physical training regime including
body building, check with a nutritionist before starting the EYY Eating Plan to
make sure your protein and carbohydrate needs are met.

Contents

Introduction 4

Five processes that age you 12
Understand the five body malfunctions that age you

Five most ageing foods 26
How to avoid the major foods that deplete your body

Five best youthing foods 42
The top five age-busters

Charting progress 62
A range of creative tests to check your progress

The EYY Detox 74
Kick-start your way to a more youthful you

The EYY Eating Plan 86
Recipes to nourish and maintain your youthfulness

Sustaining youthing for life 148
Easy ways to continue youthing for life

Recipe index 158
Acknowledgements 160

We are much more than what we eat, but what we eat can nevertheless help us be much more than what we are.

ADELLE DAVIS, NUTRITION PIONEER

Introduction

Eat Yourself Young is a practical guide to help you look, feel and live younger. Forget Botox, fillers and face-lifts – the quickest and most effective way to take years off your looks is simply by changing what you eat. That may sound unbelievable, but it's true. You can eat yourself younger, and what's more it's easier than you may think. On the **Eat Yourself Young (EYY) Programme**, you'll quickly lose weight and feel lighter, more energetic and less stressed. Your skin will improve, you'll sleep better. Soon, people will notice you are glowing with vitality. But most importantly, you'll start to look and feel younger – it's a real high when you suddenly realize it's not your age that's making you feel old, it's your food.

'A truly good doctor always tries first to cure with food,' said Chinese physician Sun Ssu-mo nearly 1,400 years ago. Food is medicine, our best-revitalizing tool, though somewhere along the way we've lost sight of that self-evident truth. On a typical day, we're more likely to be powered by supermarket sandwiches, flapjacks and copious café lattes than anything healthy. We think our bodies can handle the nutritional deprivation, and for a while perhaps they can. But as we enter our 30s and beyond, *our looks take a battering* – skin, hair and nails lose their gloss, energy levels flag and we start to look and feel worn out.

This is not a natural or inevitable part of ageing. None of us has a sell-by date imprinted in us like a stick of rock. Indeed, scientists today reject the idea that the body is programmed like a biological clock to decline in a certain way as we age. The typical symptoms of ageing are now considered to be **around 25% genetic** – with 75% from accumulated cell damage due to lifestyle and other factors.

In other words, you age the way you do largely because of the foods you eat and the lifestyle choices you make.

After years working with clients and seeing how diet improved their looks and energy levels, making them seem years younger, I became convinced that the way we age is *greatly within our control.* Indeed, many of the biological markers of age can be altered by diet, including body fat percentage, blood sugar tolerance, LDL/HDL ratio, blood pressure, the basal metabolic rate and the body's ability to regulate its internal temperature, according to the USDA Human Nutrition Research Center on Aging at Tufts University, Boston.

With this book, my aim is to bring all the youthing knowledge I've accumulated to a wider audience, and offer a new and realistic way of eating that gives everyone the power to look and feel years younger. The **EYY Programme** starts with the **How Youthful Are You?** questionnaire on pages 8–11. This gives you an idea of the functional age of your body right now, and helps you discover your youthing potential. Then I explain the *five most ageing body processes* – you can't avoid them, but I show you how to minimize their impact using good food choices – the five most ageing foods and five superfood age-busters that have a youthing effect on the body. Medical data on food has come a long way in the past 10 years and high-quality, evidence-based science now points ineradicably to the kind of foods that keep you young and healthy. It's these foods you need to incorporate into your diet on a daily basis.

The **EYY Programme** proper starts with a 2-week detox. This is a deep cleanse, and it's invaluable. By eliminating certain foods, caffeine and alcohol, your body escapes the modern-day overload of chemicals, preservatives and denatured food, and starts to *refuel with the nutritional goodies* that genuinely sustain it. Most people find that their troublesome niggles and symptoms – headaches, spots, constipation, tiredness, low mood – disappear. You become more energetic, your mind is clearer, and you feel vital and confident, able to throw off long-held habits that hold you back. The detox is a wake-up call: it helps you realize that by eating properly in a way that suits you and your lifestyle, you can reap even greater anti-ageing rewards in the future.

After detox, the **EYY Eating Plan** is a rejuvenating diet that you can follow for life. It is designed to minimize the stress caused by the five ageing processes while maximizing the intake of youthing enzymes, bioflavonoids, antioxidants, vitamins, minerals, trace elements and healthy proteins. It's based on your knowledge of the way your body operates and is flexible enough to suit *every individual's needs and tastes.* Each dish is colour-coded to ensure you get the right blend of nutrients to help the youthing process every time you sit down at the table. It's important to enjoy your food and keep excitement and adventure around mealtimes – there are around 70 exciting recipes that not only taste great, but maximize the potential in the food you eat. All use simple cooking methods that support rather than sabotage your body's functions. There is also an easy-to-use, colour-coded Youthing Food Chart (see pages 94–9) that shows you which foods pack the most powerful anti-ageing punch so you can add them into your diet.

Once you start the **EYY Programme,** you'll soon find out that the choice of ageing quickly or slowly *is in your own hands.* I can promise that within 2 weeks you'll start to feel better, within a month you'll be positive and full of energy, within 6 months you'll look at least 3–5 years younger – and within a year, well, that's up to you.

Sometimes you need to draw a line in the sand. To say that from here on, life for me will be different. This book gives you the tools to do exactly that. This is not just another diet, it's a *revolutionary journey* towards self-determination and rejuvenation, along which a leaner and more energized you will emerge. Being young is not just about your biological age: it's about feeling positive, self-confident and vibrant, about finding laughter and joy in the things you do and people you meet, about having high energy levels and a wonderful enthusiasm for life – whatever decade you happen to find yourself in.

The **EYY Programme** will not only change your body, it will change your outlook and your life. Welcome to a younger you.

WHAT DOES NORMAL AGEING LOOK LIKE

Some of the typical ageing symptoms people experience from their 30s onwards. The **EYY Programme** can slow down, and even reverse many of them.

DECADE	WOMEN	MEN
30s	Frown and nose to mouth lines appear • Slight skin thinning • Metabolism slows by about 0.5% per year • Slight loss of muscle tone • Start to lose bone mass from age 35 (at around 1% per year) • At sexual peak (from age 35 to 42) • Fertility drops (around age 37)	Start to lose muscle to fat (at rate of 3kg per decade) • Thickening around abdomen • Hair thinning and balding at crown and temples • Testosterone production in decline
40s	Crow's feet and smile lines appear (even when you're not smiling) • Jaw less defined • Waist/abdomen fat thickens • Shoulder and back fat may appear • Bottom/breasts sag • Grey hairs arrive • Face looks thinner • Less flexibility in joints, ligaments and muscles • More breathless: lose 5–10% of heart and lung capacity • Perimenopause: missed periods, headaches, mood swings, etc. • Increase in low mood (20% of women suffer depression) • Declining vision	Smile/forehead lines (men's skin is oilier than women's so lines arrive later) • Increased fat deposits on torso and around internal organs • Salt and pepper/grey temples • Balding accelerates • Slight loss of libido • Less flexibility in joints, ligaments and muscles • Decrease in stamina • More irritability, fatigue • Resting metabolism drops 2% per decade • Vision in decline
50s	Skin increasingly thinner, sallower and sags at cheek and jowl • More grey hair • Nails thicken, become ridged • Stiffer joints • Increased muscle loss • Menopause: just over half of women suffer hot flushes, night sweats, fatigue, memory loss, headaches, etc. • More fat deposited on bottom, abdomen, thighs, chin – even under eyes • Loss of energy and stamina • Loss of libido (33% of women) • Vision further declines • Increased risk of coronary heart disease/stroke • Bone thinning and osteoporosis	Deeper facial lines • sagging, thickening skin on cheeks and jowls • Grey hair and less of it • Body hair greyer • Bone mass decreases • Larger abdomen • Vision further declines • Slight height shrinkage (6mm per decade) • Higher risk of cardiovascular and circulatory diseases • Prostate enlarges (causing more frequent urination)
60s	Age spots appear • Deeper facial skin wrinkling/heavy undereye bags appear • Neck wrinkles • Skin increasingly thin and inelastic, takes longer to renew and repair • Nose and earlobes widen and lengthen • Further loss of muscle tone • Increased risk of cardiovascular disease/osteoporosis • Lower energy/stamina • Metabolic rate decreases • Body water content decreases • Decline in short-term, episodic memory	Age spots appear • Increased loss of muscle/increased body fat • Skin increasingly thin and inelastic: takes longer to repair • Thinning hair/balding accelerates • Nose and ears lengthen • Hair growth around ears/nostrils • Loss of body hair • Lower energy, stamina • Decline in short-term, episodic memory

*In order to change we must be sick
and tired of being sick and tired.*
ANON

How youthful are you?

This test helps you assess the current functional age of your body. Tick the answer that best represents your body – be truthful, it's important to get accurate ageing markers at this stage so you can compare them later and see what effect the **EYY Programme** is having over time.

Turn the page for your scores and to discover your youthing potential.

1 Food is crucial to the way you look and feel. How do you eat?

A You cook from fresh, preferably organic.

B You try to cook from fresh but eat processed foods a few times a week.

C You mostly eat pre-packaged foods, though cook once or twice a week.

D You eat out a few nights a week and often eat ready-made meals at home.

E You always eat ready meals or grab something from a coffee shop.

2 Storing fat around the abdomen can be caused by insulin-resistance or a stress-related disorder. Look at your stomach. Is it?

A Flat and firm.

B Slightly rounded with some muscle.

C Well-rounded and with bloated upper abdomen.

D Always sticks out, with rolls of fat on top.

E Carries most of your excess weight: you can barely see your toes.

3 Nails weaken and crack through dehydration, lack of keratin, vitamin C, calcium, iron, folic acid, protein or fat. Are yours?

A Strong, shiny, they rarely chip or break.

B Relatively strong, chip occasionally, no markings.

C Becoming thinner and weaker with markings.

D Grow slowly, splinter easily, thick with horizontal or vertical ridges.

E Grow slowly, snap easily, look thick, highly ridged.

4 **Your skin can become dry and thin over time. Is the skin on your forearm:**

A Silky smooth, dense and elastic? . . .   . . .

B Dense and elastic but with uneven skin tone? . . .   . . .

C Noticeably thinning with some liver spots? . . .   . . .

D Losing elasticity and looking dry, with liver spots and other discolourations? . . .   . . .

E Thin and dry, looking crepy and has lost elasticity? . . .   . . .

5 **Clear, bright eyes are a sign of youthfulness. Do yours look:**

A Clear with bright whites, and no wrinkles? . . .   . . .

B Bright, though skin on the upper eyelids is sagging a little? . . .   . . .

C Slightly yellow, with baggy upper eyelids and tiny crow's feet? . . .   . . .

D Dull, with crow's feet and loose skin around? . . .   . . .

E Dull and small, hidden in heavily creased skin? . . .   . . .

6 **Clench your buttocks, naked, and look in a mirror.
How much cellulite do you see?**

A None, area is firm and toned. . . .   . . .

B You have a bit of cellulite and a few creases. . . .   . . .

C Slightly flabby with some orange peel skin. . . .   . . .

D Fat and flabby, with orange peel all over. . . .   . . .

E Sagging with cellulite, no muscle tone. . . .   . . .

7 **Take a photo of the lower half of your face in profile. How does it look?**

A The jaw is well defined, the tip of the chin above the jawline. . . .   . . .

B Jawline is sagging a little, but chin is firm and pronounced. . . .   . . .

C Jowls are beginning to appear, chin is drooping. . . .   . . .

D There is little definition in chin and jawline is irregular. . . .   . . .

E Jawline has disappeared, you have baggy jowls. . . .   . . .

8 **Your immune system keeps you youthful by fighting off age-inducing bacteria,
bugs and viruses. How does yours function?**

A You very rarely get colds and, if you do, you get over them within 1–2 days. . . .   . . .

B You get colds twice a year and recover fairly quickly. . . .   . . .

C You get heavy colds a few times a year and find it hard to recover quickly. . . .   . . .

D You don't get sick often, but when you do, it is very serious. . . .   . . .

E You have to be careful as you seem to get sick very easily. . . .   . . .

9 **How well do you sleep? Sleep de-stresses, and is the time when your body repairs and rejuvenates.**

A You sleep well, uninterrupted and feel good when you wake up. ... ...

B You sleep well, uninterrupted but you feel groggy when you get up. ... ...

C You fall sleep easily, but wake in the night, and find it hard to get back to sleep. ... ...

D You find it hard to get to sleep, toss and turn and don't sleep that long. ... ...

E You have insomnia; you feel tired most of the time. ... ...

10 **How flexible are you? Acidification and too much sugar can cause stiff joints.**

A You can touch your toes with ease. ... ...

B You can almost touch your toes, if you warm up first. ... ...

C You cannot touch your toes but can get to your ankles. ... ...

D You can't bend over that far without fearing a strain. ... ...

E You can't bend down without bending your knees. ... ...

11 **How good is your memory? Below is a list of numbers, with ten omitted. Read them through and every time you see an omission, pause and note what number is missing (don't write it down). When you reach the end, cover the list and try to remember the missing numbers.**

1 2 3 4 5 7 8 10 11 13 14 15 16 17 19 21 22 23 24 25 27 28 30 31 32 33 35 36 38 40

A You can remember all the missing numbers correctly. ... ...

B You remember about two-thirds of them. ... ...

C You can remember about five numbers, but got a few wrong. ... ...

D You can remember two or three of the numbers, but guessed lots wrong. ... ...

E You can't remember any of them. ... ...

12 **Youthful-minded people are energetic and willing to try out new things. What is your attitude to life?**

A You feel strong, vital and enthusiastic, you like challenging yourself. ... ...

B You like change, activity and adventure, but don't get enough of it. ... ...

C You're too overwhelmed with work/family/routine to fit in anything new. ... ...

D You feel dull, sluggish, happiest with familiar friends and situations. ... ...

E You feel stuck, exhausted, fragile and frightened of change. ... ...

See opposite to read your scores

HOW YOUTHFUL ARE YOU? SCORING

Count the number of As, Bs, Cs, etc. you have ticked, then read on to discover whether your functional age – the age your body appears to be working at – reflects your real age. Once you've spent some time on the **EYY Programme**, do the questionnaire again to see your progress.

MOSTLY As

If you scored mostly As, you're in good shape. This is the youthing level of someone aged 20–30, so if you've notched up more decades than that, congratulations – you're well on the way to achieving your youthing potential. Think of the **EYY Programme** as an investment for your future: it will ease the way for you to maintain your healthy physique, mental agility and positive attitude throughout your life – to live longer, but also better. If you ticked any Cs to Fs, look on them as areas for improvement by turning them into measurable goals. Following the **EYY Programme** will make losing that inch of flab or strengthening hair, skin and nails effortlessly easy.

MOSTLY Bs

If you're over 40 and scored mostly Bs, then you are looking and feeling much younger than your chronological age. This is the youthing level of someone aged 30–40, the most crucial decade for preventative anti-ageing care. It's when people start to notice a loss of skin tone, a few wrinkles, a bit of flab around their middle. With the **EYY Programme** you can slow down these physical changes and craft a more youthful face and body for life. If you ticked any Ds or Es, these areas need immediate attention – check your symptoms in Chapters 1, 2 and 4 and make sure you eat to avoid the relevant ageing process. Although the **EYY Programme** cannot eradicate wrinkles, it can help you achieve smoother, plumper skin and a leaner body. After 2 months on the **EYY Programme**, test your scores again and see your improvements.

MOSTLY Cs

This is the youthing level of someone aged 40–50, so if you're younger than that and

ticking mostly Cs, you need to do some serious youthing work on yourself. Try the **EYY Programme** for 3 months and see how much healthier you feel. If you're aged over 50, you're doing well but there's always room for improvement. The choice of ageing quickly or slowly is in your own hands, so aim high: you want glowing skin and hair, a lean body, pots of energy and to feel positive and confident about yourself, whatever decade you happen to find yourself in. Try the **EYY Programme** for 3–6 months, then test yourself again. You'll notice remarkable changes in your body, mood, sleeping patterns and energy levels, transforming the way you look and feel.

MOSTLY Ds

This is the youthing level of someone aged 50–60, so if you ticked mostly Ds, it suggests you are currently experiencing some physical decline – perhaps loss of skin elasticity, weak nails and hair, overweight, cellulite, or the hormonal changes that occur to women and men during their 50s. These areas are all targeted on the **EYY Programme** and, by increasing nutrient-intake and avoiding the ageing body processes, you will notice drastic improvements – cellulite, for example, starts to disappear once alkalinity is improved. Try the questionnaire again after 4–6 months and see what youthing changes you can measure. Be encouraged by your improvements to look forward to an even younger you.

MOSTLY Es

If you ticked mostly Es, your current functional age is over 60. But we all know lean, fit, positive, energetic people in later life who look and act 20 years younger than their actual age and if they can do it, so can you. The **EYY Programme** will help rebalance blood sugar levels, rehydrate skin, improve alkalinity, oxygenate blood, and provide a plentiful supply of phytonutrients, antioxidants, essential minerals and vitamins, all of which help towards more youthful functioning. Try the **EYY Programme** for 4–6 months: it is designed to boost energy levels, brain functioning, memory and mood, helping you feel and look healthy, vital and as youthful as you can possibly be.

1

FIVE PROCESSES THAT AGE YOU

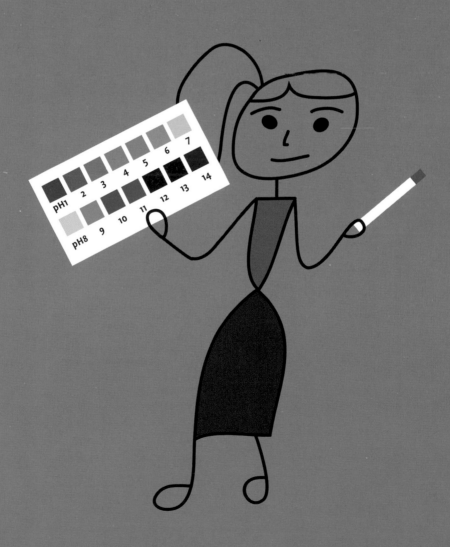

Age isn't just a number, it's your attitude to life. My aim is to help you achieve not just the physical glow of a more youthful you, but also the energy levels and sheer vitality you used to take for granted. So how can the **EYY Programme** help achieve this youthing transformation?

Working with clients, I've found there are **five normal body processes** that can get disrupted or overloaded by bad eating habits, stress or lifestyle and start to become dysfunctional. These are to do with digestion and elimination, the inflammatory response, the metabolic process called oxidation, the body's acidity/alkalinity levels, and how well the hormones are working together. When we're young, these natural processes **tick along seamlessly,** but as we grow older, the stressors can accumulate, resulting in **accelerated ageing.**

Because the processes ebb and flow interdependently, when one is under stress, it can trigger a malfunction or compensatory effect in another. For example, a sluggish bowel may lead to inflammation of the colon, fermentation of undigested food and slow elimination of toxic waste, which leads to cellular acidity and free radical damage (oxidation). In time, this negatively affects hormonal balance, an example of the five ageing processes in action.

If you don't address problems when they start, symptoms can become chronic. You may experience headaches, exhaustion, muscle/joint pains, skin wrinkling, loss of enthusiasm, lack of pleasure, and a feeling of 'old age' – even if you are only 35 years old. Diet is a major factor in **restoring the balanced functioning** of these five processes. We are what we eat, which is why I want to begin with an exploration of the five most ageing body processes, the effect they can have on your body, and how to minimize their impact using good food choices.

> **❛** Gluttony is an emotional escape,
> a sign something is eating us. **❜**
> PETER DE VRIES, NOVELIST

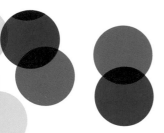

'It's not the food in your life,
it's the life in your food,
ANON

Eliminative slowdown

A well-functioning digestive system is central to the youthing process.
The gut is the engine room of the body: food goes in, nutrients are
extracted, and a neat little waste package exits the other end.
Great – until it starts underperforming.

SLOW GUT, EARLY AGEING

When the gut becomes sluggish or constIpated, the liver, kidneys, bowels, lungs and
skin are put under increased strain, causing an ageing environment in the body. Skin,
hair, nails, muscles and bones become undernourished.
Headaches, spots, chronic tiredness, low energy, high
cholesterol and depression result. That's why
**eliminative slowdown is the most important
ageing process to avoid.** Here are four
reasons why it's crucial to get your gut
working at its optimum:

> *To check your gut's
> transit time, take 5–10g
> charcoal 2 hours before eating
> and 5 hours before bed. Check how
> long it takes for your stool to come
> out black. The perfect time is 12–24
> hours. Anything more, and sluggish
> gut movement could cause toxic
> build-up. Anything less, and
> nutrients are not being
> absorbed properly.*

1 A slow eliminative system causes
wastes to accumulate, producing extra
bacteria and hormones for the liver to
process. Combine this with bad diet, stress
or antibiotics and the gut's intestinal flora
becomes unbalanced. Yeasts like candida overgrow,
producing toxic by-products, which the liver also has to
process. It becomes inefficient and the body becomes more susceptible to ageing.

2 With a sluggish gut, the body doesn't absorb nutrients, vitamins and minerals.
Hair and nails get thinner and break, skin dries and loses tone, eyes feel gritty, lose
their whiteness and may become painful, cheeks sag, weight may increase and energy
levels are depleted. You start to look and feel older.

3 A healthy gut allows nutrients to pass through its walls while blocking harmful debris. But when the gut underperforms, this debris is deposited out of the way in joints, muscles and other tissues – so-called 'leaky gut syndrome'. The immune system attacks the debris, causing an immune response that may result in joint and muscle pain, arthritis, acne, eczema and a general feeling of unwellness.

4 Around 70% of the immune system is located in the gut, so if it's sluggish, it can compromise immunity. When your immune system is stressed, you're more likely to develop infections and disorders such as food allergies and intolerances. You'll feel unwell, stress levels will rise, and the ageing process will accelerate.

IS YOUR GUT UNDER STRAIN?

If so, you may experience:

★ Bloating, belching, bad breath

★ Excessive flatulence (more than 15 times a day)

★ Sharp abdominal pains, heartburn, reflux, indigestion

★ Migraine and headache

★ Ulcerative colitis, IBS, diverticulitis, constipation, diarrhoea

★ Secondary symptoms – acne, arthritis, body odour, chronic fatigue, colds, eczema, fine lines, migraine and headache, food allergies, psoriasis.

The lining of the gut renews itself every 4–5 days, so improvement is possible – fast!

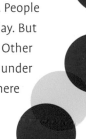

PERFECT POOPING

A healthy stool should look like a smooth banana with a point at one end, well-hydrated and with no mucus on it. If yours looks like rabbit droppings or compacted balls wadded together, it has been sitting in the colon for too long. People often don't realize they are constipated – especially if they pass a stool every day. But if your faecal matter is hard or difficult to expel, you are probably constipated. Other telltale physical signs are fine horizontal lines on the forehead and baggy skin under the eyes. Press on the inside of your left hip: your stool builds up in the colon here and discomfort/bloating/gas is often a sign of sluggish elimination.

THE GUT/MOOD CONNECTION

The digestive system contains more neurons than the spinal cord and more neurotransmitters than the brain – 90% of serotonin is created in the bowels, so a sluggish gut *influences mood* and *emotional wellbeing* too. You'll have more energy and positivity once your bowel movements are sorted out.

See pages 94–9 for foods that will combat eliminative slowdown.

'Age is a case of mind over matter.
If you don't mind, it don't matter,'

SATCHEL PAIGE, US BASEBALL PLAYER

Inflammation

Inflammation is our fast, natural response to injury, allergy and infection – as soon as a splinter pierces your skin, the inflammatory response kicks in to protect you. As we age, this everyday response can become over-reactive – scientists have coined the word 'inflammaging' to describe the state of chronic, low-level inflammation in the body.

Research shows **inflammation is a root cause of wrinkles and muscle loss,** as well as diseases such as inflammatory bowel, rheumatoid arthritis, diabetes, stroke, cancer and Alzheimer's. But how can the body's natural healing response have such a negative effect? It works like this. Whether you've *cut your finger* or been exposed to a *cold virus,* a cascade of events is set in motion called the inflammatory response. On the surface, you'll notice swelling, redness and pain. Behind the scenes, the immune system's white blood cells neutralize the threat, then the inflammatory trigger is switched off and **tissue repair begins.** The problem comes when the inflammatory response isn't fully switched off and the body stays inflamed. Activated immune cells circulate in the bloodstream, causing a series of molecular and cellular changes, which take a heavy toll on the body. Irritants such as food additives, exposure to household chemicals or stress may start to trigger excessive inflammatory reactions.

Some women first notice joint pain and other inflammatory symptoms during the menopause, when oestrogen levels drop. Eating a diet rich in plant oestrogens (beans, seeds, leafy greens, wholegrains) helps lessen inflammation naturally.

As the immune system becomes more unbalanced, the effects spiral, resulting in infections, allergies, loss of skin quality and other ageing signs. Sometimes immune cells attack healthy tissues, causing autoimmune diseases such as rheumatoid arthritis. That's why reducing inflammation is a **crucial step to successful youthing.**

ARE YOU INFLAMED?

With chronic, low-grade inflammation, you may experience:

★ Allergies/food intolerances, acne, eczema, hives and rashes

★ Diarrhoea/colitis/mucus on the stool

★ Dry eyes, fatigue, gas, indigestion

★ Fine lines

★ Night eating

★ Headaches/restless leg syndrome

★ Frequent colds/infections/congestion/mucus

★ Joint pain/stiffness, loss of skin firmness/elasticity

★ Swelling/bloating, especially in your hands and feet

> Stay away from foods that make your nose run, eyes water or cause bloating – these are inflammatory responses!

HOW TO AVOID INFLAMMATION

★ Lower your unrefined sugar intake

★ Stay away from foods you know you are allergic to

★ Don't eat too much of any one food group – protein, fat or carbs

★ Eat organic where you can to avoid chemical additives and preservatives

★ Avoid alcohol

★ Keep your gut healthy (see pages 14–5)

★ Keep your body alkaline (see pages 20–3)

★ Keep stress levels as low as possible and try to avoid getting depressed (both cause inflammatory markers in the blood)

★ Avoid taking NSAIDs (non-steroidal anti-inflammatory drugs), such as ibuprofen, for minor ailments on a frequent basis as it may irritate the gut lining.

EAT ANTI-INFLAMMATORY

The immune system starts in the gut so if it's inflamed (signs are gas, bloating, loose stools, tenderness), your immunity is compromised, meaning you cannot turn off the inflammatory response. What you eat is crucial to rebalancing your body – one study of overweight people showed that just 1 week after starting a nutritious diet, levels of inflammation dropped. The **EYY Eating Plan** is designed to help soothe inflammation by boosting your intake of foods containing inflammation-dampening antioxidants called polyphenols, which includes curcumin (see pages 48–51), and omega-3 fatty acids, and helping you stay off inflammatory foods such as sugar, white flour, red meat and some dairy products.

See pages 94–9 for foods that will help you fight inflammation.

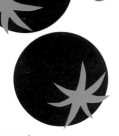

'Tell me what you eat,
and I will tell you what you are,'

JEAN ANTHELME BRILLAT-SAVARIN, GASTRONOME

Oxidation

Oxygen is the basis of life. It creates energy and is crucial in most of the metabolic functions that keep us alive. Each of the trillions of cells in our bodies need a constant supply of oxygen and nutrients to work properly and help us stay energetic and vital. But oxygen is also dangerous: just as an apple turns brown on contact with air, the oxidation process can lead to cellular toxicity and damage, resulting in accelerated signs of ageing, including the early onset of wrinkles, loss of skin elasticity, muscle tone and low energy levels.

Oxygen is a **highly reactive chemical,** always looking to combine with other molecules it meets. These chemical reactions create 'free radicals' – unstable atoms with an unpaired electron (a negatively charged particle) in their outer layer. To stabilize themselves, they 'steal' electrons from other compounds, thus creating more free radicals, which then steal more electrons ... and so on. This destructive cascade can eventually cause what scientists call '*oxidative stress*' and the theft of electrons from atoms within cell membranes, proteins, lipids and genes. Prolonged oxidative stress can damage cell structure, and even DNA and RNA – your body's genetic building block and the messaging service it relies on.

Did you know: although free radicals can be destructive, they also perform many useful jobs – they act as cellular messengers, attack bacteria and help transform food into energy, for example.

ANTIOXIDANTS TO THE RESCUE

Although the body has evolved many defences to protect itself against oxidative stress, it can become overwhelmed when external toxins such as cigarette smoke,

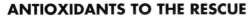

alcohol, recreational drugs, stress, overweight, UV light, chemicals in foods and household cleaning products, add to the load. That's when diet can help. Colourful foods contain high levels of antioxidants – the vitamins, polyphenols and other phytonutrients that neutralize free radicals by giving up an electron to bond with them. You could say that antioxidants sacrifice themselves to protect other important molecules from damage. Major antioxidants include vitamins C and E; carotenoids such as lycopene and lutein; polyphenols such as flavonoids and resveratrol; and the minerals selenium and zinc, which help process the antioxidant enzymes needed to neutralize free radicals.

There is accumulating evidence that **boosting antioxidants in the diet increases what scientists call 'functional lifespan'** – how well your body operates, which is the basis of the youthing process. By eating a diet rich in antioxidants, you can protect yourself from oxidative stress, minimize cellular damage and *promote youthing and high energy levels* – whatever your biological age.

EAT COLOUR

Look at your plate – if it is full of dark brown and white foods, then you are not getting the range of antioxidants you need. Go for highly coloured fruit, veg and whole foods at every meal – studies show that black, red and brown chickpeas contain 30 times the antioxidant activity of beige ones, and that red and purple-skinned potatoes contain more than twice the antioxidants of tan-skinned ones. Colours to eat are:

★ **Green and dark green,** such as kale, spinach, celery, courgettes, kiwi fruit
★ **Yellow and orange,** such as lemons, carrots, sweet potatoes, squash, apricots
★ **Red,** such as tomatoes, watermelon, red beans
★ **Yellowy brown,** such as wheatgerm, nuts, seeds, vegetable oils
★ **Blue/purple,** such as aubergines, beetroot, blackberries, blueberries, figs, purple grapes
★ **Tawny red/black,** such as cacao nibs, green tea, dark chocolate (in moderation, please!).

See pages 94–9 for more antioxidant foods.

Eat more orange and yellow veg and fruit! After 2 months, skin takes on a lightly tanned, just-back-from-skiing glow that looks very youthing.

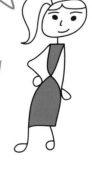

> 'Rich, fatty foods are like destiny:
> they too shape our ends.'
>
> ANON

Acidification

One of the body's most important ongoing jobs is to balance the levels of acidity and alkalinity in the cells. Everything functions better when intracellular fluid is in a slightly alkaline state, at a pH of around 7.2–7.4 (with pH 7 as neutral). That's when there's a plentiful supply of antioxidants, anti-ageing phytonutrients, essential minerals and vitamins to encourage youthful functioning. Bones are strong and the kidneys and liver detoxify efficiently. Fungi and candida find it hard to take hold; sugar cravings diminish; and inflammation and degenerative diseases are kept at bay.

When you eat a meal high in acid-forming foods, balance it later in the day with a big glass of green juice. Try a mix of celery, spinach, lettuce, kale, parsley, lemon and fresh ginger. It'll boost your alkalinity.

In an optimum alkaline state, you start to feel young again, full of energy, with strong muscles and good coordination, smooth skin, sleek hair and bright eyes. But how does your body maintain this happy alkaline state? Mostly it's about what you eat. Diet has a powerful effect on the body's acid-alkaline balance. We tend to *consume too many acid-producing foods,* such as meat, fish, grains, cheese, eggs, cereals, sweet drinks, sugary snacks, alcohol and coffee. This can result in a long-term acid overload, called acidification, which changes the body's environment and makes it susceptible to destructive ageing processes.

The more acidic the body, the quicker wrinkles are formed, skin dries and cracks, nails thin and splinter, hair dulls and falls out. To buffer excess acid, minerals such as calcium and magnesium are pulled from the bones, weakening them and potentially leading to osteoporosis. A build-up of uric acid in the system may cause

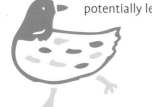
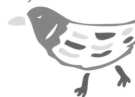

joint stiffness, gout and osteoarthritis. Iodine is taken from soft tissue, negatively affecting the thyroid and leading to *fatigue, depression,* mental slowing, weight gain and diabetes. Chronic acidity encourages fatty acids to go from a negative to a positive charge and stick to artery walls, increasing the risk of diabetes and heart disease. Enzyme function weakens, leading to digestive disorders, food allergies and an inability to repair damaged tissue. In an acidic body, the attack from outside as well as the pathogens from within become overwhelming and it is this that creates long-term damage and degenerative malfunctioning.

There is a big difference between acidic foods and acid-forming foods – for example, although lemon juice is acidic, it has an alkalizing effect in the body, as it metabolizes to an alkaline 'citrate'. The same is true of other citrus fruits.

THE PERFECT BALANCE

It's easy to see why avoiding acidification is one of my top youthing priorities. By changing your diet to incorporate more alkaline than acid-forming foods, you can *reverse acidity* and take your body into a youthing alkaline state. Alkaline foods such as vegetables, fruits and legumes are **intrinsically healthy,** full of minerals, vitamins, amino acids, enzymes, immune enhancers and phytochemicals (see the chart overleaf). **Aim to eat 80% alkaline to 20% acid-forming foods** to reverse acidification, then keep levels stable by eating a balance of no less than 70%/30%. Hard cheeses, meats and animal fats are highly acid-forming and hard for the body to process, so avoid them and eat more easily processed proteins such as vegetable protein, legumes and yoghurts instead.

THE ACID TEST

How can you tell if your body is over-acidic? One way is to check the pH of your urine.

★ Run a pH test strip or litmus paper (from chemists, health food shops or online) in your early morning urine for a couple of seconds.

★ Compare the colour reading to the chart.

★ The pH of urine can range from highly acid (4.5) to alkaline (8), but a healthy reading will be slightly **acid, around pH 6.4–6.8** (morning urine is more acidic).

★ If your pH is too acid (below 6), aim to rebalance your system by eating more alkaline foods.

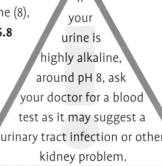

If your urine is highly alkaline, around pH 8, ask your doctor for a blood test as it may suggest a urinary tract infection or other kidney problem.

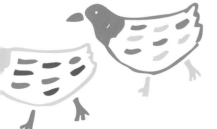
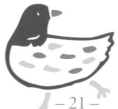

ALKALINE AND ACIDIC FOODS

FOODS	ACID	WEAK ACIDS
SWEETENERS	Aspartame, barley malt syrup, brown rice syrup, brown sugar, corn syrup, fructose, milk and most other chocolate, milk sugar, processed honey, refined sugar, white sugar	Agave syrup, malt, maple syrup, molasses, raw honey, 90% dark chocolate
DAIRY & ALTERNATIVES	Butter, cow's milk, cream, custard, hard cheeses, homogenized milk, ice cream, margarine, Quark	Cottage cheese, cow's milk sweetened yoghurt
FATS & OILS	Goose fat, lard, peanut oil, pistachio oil, walnut oil, safflower oil	Corn oil, nut butters
MEAT & EGGS	All meats, meat products (e.g. dried meats, gelatine, sausages), game, poultry	Eggs – any varieties
FISH	All seafood, smoked/cured fish	Fresh fish
GRAINS	Corn, corn flakes, cornmeal, white refined flour, white rice	Brown rice, oats, spelt, wholegrain wheat
FRUIT	Tinned fruit	Blackcurrant/red/pink/white, cranberries, damsons, gooseberries
VEGETABLES		Broad/fava beans, mushrooms: button, garden, portobello
LEGUMES		Chickpeas, haricot verts, lentils, split peas
NUTS & SEEDS		Brazil, cashew, macadamia, peanut (unsalted), pecan, pistachio, walnut
HERBS & SPICES		
DRINKS	Black tea, coffee, fizzy drinks, fruit juices from concentrate, soft drinks, beer, cider, spirits, wine (red and white)	Fresh fruit juices (except lemon and lime), Champagne, fruit tea, mature organic red and white wine
OTHER	Additives, E-numbers, preservatives, processed foods	Balsamic vinegar, wine vinegar

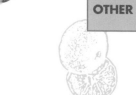

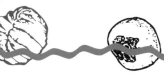

See pages 94–9 for more alkaline foods.

MILDLY ALKALINE	ALKALINE	FOODS
Sweet apricot paste, xylitol		**SWEETENERS**
Bio yoghurt, buttermilk, goat/sheep/ buffalo's products (cheese, yoghurt and milk), kefir, whey	Almond milk, cashew milk, coconut milk, hazelnut milk, sesame milk (unsweetened), soya cheese and milk	**DAIRY & ALTERNATIVES**
Coconut oil, hazelnut oil, olive oil, pumpkin oil, rapeseed oil, seed butters, sesame oil, sunflower oil	Almond oil, avocado oil, borage oil, flaxseed/linseed oil, grapeseed oil	**FATS & OILS**
		MEAT & EGGS
		FISH
Amaranth, barley (pearl), black/red rice, buckwheat, quinoa, rye	Chickpea, lentil or soya flour, millet, soy lecithin, sprouted grains, wheatgerm	**GRAINS**
Apple, banana, beansprouts, most berries, cherry, goji berry, grapefruit, guava, olive, orange, peach/nectarine, raspberry, strawberry, tomato	Avocado, date, fig, grape, kiwi fruit, lemon, lime, mango, melon, papaya, passion fruit, pear, pineapple, plum, raisin, watermelon	**FRUIT**
Asparagus, aubergine, beetroot green tops, broccoli, chicory, mushroom (shiitake), onion, pepper (bell, sweet), potato, rocket, spring onion, sweetcorn	Artichoke, barley grass, beetroot (fresh), cabbage (all kinds), carrot, courgette, cucumber, endive, fennel, garlic, green beans, leek, lettuce, peas, pumpkin, radish, spinach, squash, swede, sweet potato, turnip, watercress, wheatgrass	**VEGETABLES**
Most beans, including aduki, black, miso, pinto, small red and soya/edamame, tempeh/tofu	Alfalfa sprouts	**LEGUMES**
Almonds, chestnuts, coconut, hazelnuts, pumpkin seeds, sunflower seeds, tahini	Caraway seeds, cumin seeds, fennel seeds, flaxseeds/linseeds, sesame seeds	**NUTS & SEEDS**
	All herbs and spices, including basil, chilli, chives, cinnamon, coriander, curry leaf, dill, ginger, horseradish, mustard, nutmeg, oregano, parsley, rosemary, turmeric	**HERBS & SPICES**
Soda water	Coconut water, distilled water, filtered water, herbal teas (the fresher the better), lemon and lime juice, veg juices	**DRINKS**
Bovril, Marmite, miso, Vegemite	Apple cider vinegar (with mother)	**OTHER**

'Life isn't about finding yourself.
Life is about creating yourself.'

GEORGE BERNARD SHAW, PLAYWRIGHT

Hormonal imbalance

Hormones have a direct impact on your appearance, activity levels, and the way you feel about yourself. These chemical messengers are great youthing helpers – when your hormones are balanced you'll have clear, glowing skin, glossy hair and nails, and a lean body. But when you are hormonally unbalanced, your body is on an anti-youthing rollercoaster – you put on weight, your skin starts to wrinkle, you sleep badly, feel stressed, and begin to look much older than your years.

YOUTHING HORMONES

For youthing, the most important hormones are insulin, the stress hormones adrenaline and cortisol, and the thyroid hormones, which control metabolism. These hormones are affected by diet, especially the intake of carbohydrates and fats. The sex hormones (oestrogen, progesterone, testosterone) also have powerful youthing potential. As well as dictating the way your body reacts during puberty, the menstrual cycle, pregnancy, the menopause, andropause (male menopause) and beyond, **they help keep skin, bone, joints, connective tissue and teeth healthy and strong.** The effects caused by an imbalance of these sex hormones can be minimized by diet.

When your hormones are balanced, you'll enjoy that most youthful of all feelings, energy!

HORMONAL IMBALANCE: THE SYMPTOMS

With hormones, we tend to think about monthly mood swings. But hormones aren't just about sex – these chemical substances work non-stop to keep almost every body system functioning. They regulate temperature, make sure muscles and brain are supplied with food, control appetite, blood sugar, metabolism, where you store fat and how easily you lose it. They *affect mood* and *counterbalance stress* to help you sleep well and keep calm and focused.

Imbalance of the stress hormones adrenaline and cortisol may cause: wrinkles, abdominal fat gain, sleep disturbances, anxiety, mood swings, allergies, headaches, susceptibility to infection, muscle weakness, sugar/alcohol cravings, gas and bloating, heart palpitations, lack of testosterone and libido.

Imbalance of the thyroid hormones may cause: fatigue, dry skin, heart palpitations, cold hands and feet, thinning hair, brittle nails, constipation, weight gain/inability to lose weight, menstrual irregularities, loss of libido.

Too much insulin may cause: cellulite, sagging skin, abdominal fat, fast weight gain, fatigue, poor memory, carb cravings, disrupted sleep, mood disorders, elevated blood fats, insulin resistance, diabetes.

WOMEN'S TESTOSTERONE DECLINES DURING MENOPAUSE, LEADING TO LESS MUSCLE AND EVEN MORE FAT AROUND THE MIDDLE. EAT LOTS OF CABBAGE AND BROCCOLI – GOOD TESTOSTERONE-SUPPORTING FOODS (BUT DON'T EAT BRASSICAS IF YOU HAVE LOW THYROID).

YOUTHING BALANCE

Because hormones counterbalance each other in a highly complex way, a long-term deficiency or overproduction of a specific hormone, often caused by bad diet or high levels of stress, can cause others to over-react. The healthy, well-balanced diet you'll eat on the **EYY Programme** helps you take control of your hormones whatever stage of life you're at. Your insulin levels will stabilize, hormonally induced mood swings, anxiety and depression will ease. Lowering your stress levels with good food and sleep will affect mood, libido and sex hormones – boosting your sex drive. Once these are balanced, they, in turn, regulate the thyroid hormones. With these working in harmony, your body will be running smoothly, *able to fulfil its youthing potential.*

YOUTHING YOUR BELLY FAT

If you have hard-to-shift belly fat, it's probably because of excess levels of insulin and cortisol. Too much insulin (triggered by eating too many sugary foods) encourages unused glucose to be laid down as abdominal fat and prevents your body using that fat for energy. Excess cortisol (caused by stress, including hunger and worry) draws on muscle instead of fat for fuel, causing the loss of calorie-burning muscle and further slowing metabolism. Both hormones also increase appetite and make you crave comfort foods high in carbs and fat – which are also laid down in the abdomen. It's a vicious cycle but balancing your hormones by eating the **EYY** way can break it.

See pages 94–9 for foods that will help hormone imbalance.

2

FIVE MOST AGEING FOODS

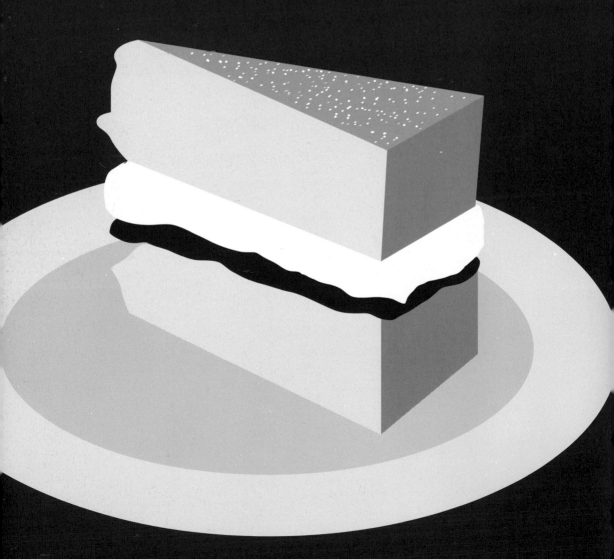

What makes a food delicious, the fat or flavour, saltiness or sweetness, the creamy rich 'mouth feel' or the 'bliss point', that perfect moment when we want more, more, more? Interestingly, it is all of these. **Our taste buds and brains are highly attuned to flavour – especially to sugar and salt** – but also to the texture, smoothness and satisfaction that certain foods provide.

That's where food manufacturers have us twisted in knots. They design foods high in sugar, salt, bad fats and nutritionally dubious additives **to satisfy our complex taste/brain needs.** These foods give us such pleasure that we eat them instead of healthy, more natural foods. And that is supremely anti-youthing, because it deprives us of the nutritional benefits we need for tiptop functioning.

Other foods we love – including meat and milk – may also be hard for the body to tolerate. They often contain pesticides and hormones, which add to their anti-youthing load and trigger the five ageing processes we're aiming to minimize. Yet somehow we think of them as healthy staples we can't live without.

This chapter goes behind the myths to help you understand which foods age you and why. Once you've read it, take a deep breath and imagine yourself giving up these delicious foods. It will feel like a tragedy, denying yourself for the sake of – what? A leaner body, fresher, youthful skin, an optimistic outlook, great sleep and bags of energy. Is it worth it? That's a choice that ultimately only you can make. But be heartened: **a few weeks** after changing their diet, studies show people often lose the cravings for junk, sweet, salty and high-fat foods, which means **the youthing dice will be loaded in your favour.**

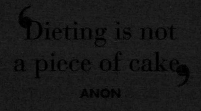

'Dieting is not
a piece of cake'
ANON

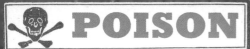 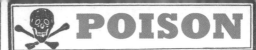 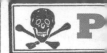

> '*Stressed spelled backwards is desserts. Coincidence? I think not.*'
>
> **ANON**

Sugar

Sugar is one of my five most ageing foods. That sounds extraordinary, as every cell in the body needs glucose to survive. The brain would starve and die without it, and our muscles would waste away. But there's a vast difference between simple sugars – the refined or processed kind usually added to foods – and the slow-releasing carbohydrates that the body converts to glucose for use as fuel. One is ageing, the other is vital and necessary, and in the right amounts will keep the brain and body young and fit.

The trouble with refined sugar is that it's addictive. It's been found to trigger the same pleasure receptors in the brain as heroin.

IT MAKES US FEEL SATISFIED AND RELAXED,

IT MAKES US WANT MORE!

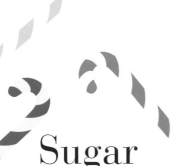

Sugar has been shown to shorten lifespan. When US biochemist Professor Cynthia Kenyon gave it to lab roundworms she'd genetically tweaked to live much longer than normal, she found it dramatically shortened their lives. She has eradicated processed sugars from her diet – and 'feels like a kid again'.

Today, refined and hidden sugars are almost impossible to avoid. They are added to processed and tinned foods, breakfast cereals, breads, cakes, biscuits, sweets and fizzy drinks. Worryingly, *now even healthy foods are sweetened.* Hummus and veg dips are 'caramelized'; peanuts and almonds are honey-roasted; supermarket apples, grapes, pineapples and sweetcorn varieties are bred to be 'super sweet'; 'crunchy' mueslis have added glucose or corn syrup; even chilli sauce has miraculously become 'sweet' chilli sauce.

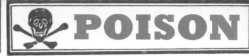
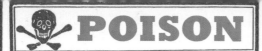

Sugar is involved in three of the ageing processes: it can create acidity, cause inflammation and disturb the hormonal balance of the body. If you drink alcohol and fruit juice and eat processed foods, then your blood sugar levels will almost certainly be too high. In youthing terms, this is catastrophic. Eating a diet full of highly sugared foods **slows the body's ability to regenerate itself** and so speeds the ageing process. On a daily level it causes – well, have a look at the list below. Excessive consumption interferes with insulin response – the hormone that tells your body to pull excess glucose from the blood and store it for later use as fat – and **can trigger a range of serious degenerative diseases** including diabetes, heart disease, osteoporosis and arthritis.

Sugar has been shown to shorten lifespan, hence its nickname – the 'white death'. Refined sugar contains no vitamins, minerals, proteins nor fibre, in fact, no nutritional elements at all. Just a lot of calories. *It's the most ageing food of all,* and one of the first steps of the **EYY Programme** is to reverse the damage it causes. By ditching refined sugars and eating slow-release complex carbohydrates (from wholegrains, pulses, vegetables and fruit) instead, you'll stabilize your long-term blood sugar levels and gain the optimum fuel for your body. The knock-on effects? You'll nourish and repair your system, have better resistance to age-related illnesses, and experience **increased motivation, energy and vitality.** It is the passport to making yourself feel years younger. Like a kid again.

YOUTH PROOF YOUR BRAIN

Your brain runs on glucose. It's the **fuel for hungry brain cells** (which use twice as much energy as other cells). Glucose helps you *focus, remember and learn.* But because the brain, unlike other organs, cannot store glucose, the amount it gets is the amount that happens to be travelling round the bloodstream at any one time. This makes it supremely vulnerable to fluctuating levels of blood sugar. So, wolfing down a sugary snack or fizzy drink is like injecting your brain with glucose. You get an instant hit, which quickly diminishes, and your brain goes into crisis mode. You feel weak, shaky, headachey, moody and unable to concentrate. In short, all the ageing symptoms of hypoglycaemia. The answer is to **avoid processed sugars and fuel your brain with complex carbohydrates instead.**

✴ ✴ ✴
AGEING EFFECTS OF 'BAD' SUGARS

★ Aching joints
★ Cravings
★ Flabby belly
★ Inability to lose weight easily
★ Lack of muscle tone
★ Lowered mental alertness
★ Mood swings
★ Puffy eyes
★ Sagging skin
★ Sluggishness
★ Spots and acne
★ Tooth decay
★ Weight gain
★ Wrinkles and lines
✴ ✴ ✴

GETTING SWEETNESS INTO YOUR LIFE

How do you get sweetness in your diet when you don't add refined sugar, honey or other sweeteners to your food? *It's easier than you think.* So many foods contain natural sugars and are intensely sweet. For example:

★ Use dried dates or apricots – see Sweet Apricot Paste (see page 145) – in puddings instead of sugar to give a natural sweetness.

★ For a sweet sauce, mix the juice of an orange, lemon, bit of ginger and half a pear and pour over fruit salads – it enhances the flavour and intensifies the sweetness of the fruits.

★ Liquorice is around 50 times sweeter than sugar: chewing on the root once a week soothes any sugary cravings and – even better – helps protect against tooth decay (though don't use if you have high blood pressure).

★ Lots of savoury foods are sweet too: try beetroot, carrots, sweet potato, tomato, almonds or pistachios when you're craving a sweet kick.

★ Adding dried fenugreek or cinnamon to your carbohydrates helps slow down the sugar rush by balancing blood sugar levels and regulating insulin.

★ Blending homemade fruit juice with flax, pumpkin, sunflower, sesame or hemp seeds will stop the fructose (fruit sugar) from entering your bloodstream quickly, as good fats slow down the metabolism of sugar.

★ If you have fat around your middle, cut down on your sugar intake – including fruit sugars. Although fruit has great antioxidant and youthing benefits, eaten in large quantities it does not do your insulin levels or belly fat any good. *One piece a day is enough* while you are regulating your insulin levels. The best slow-release sugars to eat are quinoa, pearl barley, sprouted breads, buckwheat, oatmeal, amaranth, millet and wholegrains.

SUGAR SCIENCE

Excessive intake of 'refined' sugars **causes destruction in the body.** Breaking them down involves a high-risk process called glycation, which has serious side effects. The excess glucose fuses with proteins in the muscles, skin and other organs, releasing massive amounts of damaging free radicals and what's known as 'advanced glycation end products' (AGEs) in the process. AGEs can destroy collagen, the protein that helps keep skin firm, connective tissue strong and muscles toned. The result is sagging skin, weak muscles, stiff joints, low energy and diminishing eyesight and hearing. People think this physical deterioration is a natural, normal part of the ageing process – not true! *Much of it is sugar-related.* Teenagers who eat high loads of sugar are accelerating the ageing process with every mouthful just as much as someone in their 40s!

ADDED SUGARS

Processed sugars are often added to foodstuffs, soft drinks, breads and cereals to make them more palatable. Look on food labels and avoid the following wherever you can: barley malt, beet sugar, dextrose (commercial glucose), galactose, glucose, glucose-fructose syrup/corn syrup, invert sugar, lactose, liquid fructose, maltodextrin, maltose, malt syrup, maple syrup (mostly sucrose), refined honey (to which sugar has been added), rice syrup, sorbitol and sucrose (table sugar).

SUGAR SURPRISES

Did you know that:

★ Almost everything you put into your mouth contains sugar or will break down into sugar once it is in your body? Sugar is to be found in grains, dairy products, vegetables, fruits and wine – so even if you abstain from chocolate bars and doughnuts, don't be fooled into thinking you have a low sugar diet.

★ All sugar substitutes, including aspartame, saccharin and sucralose, give your liver a lot of extra work and can cause unpleasant side effects? If you need a sweet treat, a few squares of good-quality 80% chocolate is a better youthing option.

★ Rice cakes are full of sugar? People think they are a healthy snack, but they are highly refined and pump sugar into the bloodstream as fast as eating a slice of cake. Avoid them. *As a rule of thumb:* if a food no longer looks like its original form, such as rice cakes, then don't eat it – it will be so denatured your body won't know how to process it easily.

To beat sugar cravings, eat a bit of protein instead – try nuts, cheese, soya/edamame beans or tofu.

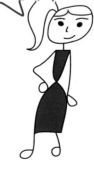

'My doctor said I looked like a million dollars – all green and wrinkled,'

RED SKELTON, COMEDIAN

Salt

Salt – that's sodium chloride – occurs naturally in many healthy foods including veg, herbs, grains, fish and meat. Sodium and chloride are important mineral salts that, along with potassium, work in balance to keep muscles, nerves and cells functioning at their best. So why is this natural, essential compound such an ageing food? Because today it is almost impossible not to eat too much of it – and over-consumption causes four of the five ageing processes to accelerate (see how, below).

BIG, BAD ANTI-YOUTHER

One of the most youthing steps you can take is to cut extra salt from your diet now. You'll notice the difference in glowing looks, better body functioning and higher energy levels (to say nothing of lower blood pressure too).

A high-salt diet causes inflammation: the cells swell with water which upsets the sodium/potassium balance that generates the energy needed to move muscles and nerves, causing weakness and fatigue.

Salt is ubiquitous in highly processed foods: it works as a cheap flavour enhancer and preservative so is added to crisps, savoury snacks, ready meals and fast foods. But it's also found in 'healthy' foods like cottage cheese, bran cereals, vegetable juices, tinned fish, cheeses, bottled olives, canned beans, hams and cold meats, soups, condiments and pickles. In fact, 80% of our daily salt intake comes from eating manufactured foods (that is anything in a box, tin or package) – and we don't need it.

Salt causes acidity, which pulls calcium from the bones – the symptoms are dry skin, brittle nails, stiff joints, calcium deposits on fingers and toes, and loss of healthy bone. *It can affect digestion* by irritating the stomach lining and reducing the production of the digestive enzyme pepsin, causing duodenal and gastric ulcers. It may also *unbalance the complex hormonal system,* causing adrenal stress, thyroid imbalance and insulin resistance. One Finnish study shows that high salt intake is associated with an increased risk of type 2 diabetes. Eating salty foods is also *highly addictive* and makes you thirsty – often for soft, carbonated drinks. So you end up eating and drinking more sweet high calorie foods and pile on the weight. The good news is that lessening salt intake while eating more fruit and veg can shift your body to a healthy youthing balance.

HOW MUCH SALT A DAY?

Most adults in Britain eat 8.6g salt a day, but you should cut back your intake to no more than 3g salt (that's around 1g sodium) a day. The easy way to do this is to stop eating processed foods with more than 0.2g sodium per 100g. Second, stop adding salt to foods you cook or eat. Be aware that even foods claiming to be 'salt-free' can contain up to 5mg salt per 100g.

HIDDEN SALTS

Sodium goes under many names. On labels look out for baking powder, bicarbonate of soda, monosodium glutamate, sodium alginate (in ice creams), sodium benzoate (in pickles, dressings, carbonated drinks), sodium chloride, sodium hydroxide (in pretzels, olives), sodium nitrite (in cured meats) and sodium sulphite (in dried fruits).

* * *

AGEING EFFECTS OF TOO MUCH SALT

★ Dry, lined skin
★ Fatigue
★ High blood pressure
★ Kidney stress
★ Loss of bone mass
★ Lowered libido
★ Muscle weakness
★ Nervous tension/anxiety
★ PMT and menstrual disorders
★ Prostate problems
★ Sore, cracked lips
★ Thinning hair
★ Tooth decay
★ Water retention and swelling
★ Weight problems

* * *

If you give up salt for 5 days, then have something salty like crisps, you instantly feel your body responding negatively to it.

YOUTHING SALT

Instead, spice up your food with basil, thyme, mint, cumin, lemon, garlic, nutmeg or pepper. If you must have a little salt, use unrefined, traditionally harvested salt such as Himalayan rock salt or Celtic sea salt. They contain ten or more mineral ions, which help nerve and muscle function, compared to table salt, which only has two. They also taste much saltier, so you need less.

'Age is something that doesn't matter, unless you are a cheese.'

BILLIE BURKE, ACTOR

Cow's dairy

We tend to think of milk (by which I mean cow's milk) as a wonder food that provides much of the calcium, vitamins and protein we need. But cow's milk products knock the body's youthing efforts for six. They trigger four of the ageing processes (see below) as well as being high in fat, cholesterol and calories, they lack many essential minerals and phytonutrients, and are often full of toxins including artificial hormones, antibiotics and pesticides. Increasing evidence suggests cow's dairy may be linked with serious health problems including osteoporosis, obesity, diabetes, some cancers and heart disease. It's no surprise that it's best avoided.

COW'S MILK IS THE PERFECT FOOD FOR BABY COWS: IT CONTAINS ALL THE NATURAL GROWTH HORMONE, NUTRIENTS AND ANTIBODIES THEY NEED.

But it's not so good for humans. It can be a major allergen, affect blood sugar and increase levels of insulin and oestrogen, causing a hormonal imbalance. Studies show that children fed cow's milk at an early age are more likely to develop asthma, eczema, digestive disorders, constipation, milk allergy and even type 1 diabetes.

Milk can affect digestion especially badly – worldwide around 75% (and in Britain up to 15%) of people lack the lactase enzyme, which processes lactose, the naturally occurring sugar in milk. As a result they suffer chronic bloating, constipation, diarrhoea, wind and nausea. Nutrients aren't absorbed properly, the undigested lactose ferments, producing gases and irritating the gut. This may kick off a chronic immune response, changing the balance of bacterial flora, and disrupting the permeability of the gut – all of which cause signs of accelerated ageing.

Gut irritation *sets off inflammation,* which may trigger mucus, stiff joints and inflammatory bowel disorders such as ulcerative colitis as well. The liver becomes overtaxed and underperforms, dumping the toxins it can't process in fat stores as cellulite.

Finally, *milk is acid-forming* so needs to be counterbalanced with lots of alkalizing foods such as vegetables – otherwise calcium leaches from bones and teeth, negating the effect of eating this so-called calcium-rich food in the first place!

On the **EYY Programme,** you will notice a big difference when you stop eating cow's dairy and substitute plant youthers for calcium instead (see below). And if you must have a bit of dairy, eat goat/sheep/buffalo's milk products instead: they are richer in many vitamins and minerals, contain anti-inflammatory oligosaccharides, which boost friendly gut bacteria, and have smaller fat globules, so are much easier to digest (especially yoghurt and kefir, which are already fermented).

> ★ ★ ★
> ## AGEING EFFECTS OF 'BAD' SUGARS
> ★ Acne and pus-filled spots
> ★ Asthma and ezcema
> ★ Bone loss and osteoporosis
> ★ Cellulite
> ★ Constipation and digestive disorders
> ★ Gas
> ★ Low energy
> ★ Sniffles and mucus
> ★ Stiff joints
> ★ Weight gain
> ★ Wrinkles
> ★ ★ ★

PLANT YOUTHERS

These plant foods come ready mixed with all of the minerals and vitamins you need to maximize calcium absorption:

Dark leafy greens: broccoli, cabbage, kale, spinach, beet greens, pak choi, plus avocado, okra.

Beans: aduki beans, black-eyed beans, chickpeas, lentils, mangetout, pinto beans, soya/edamame beans, tofu.

Nuts and seeds: almond, Brazil, flaxseed, hazelnut, pecan, pistachio, sesame, sunflower, walnut, tahini, nut butters.

Nut milks such as almond, cashew and coconut are delicious in drinks, smoothies, on porridge and cereals (for recipe, see page 147).

Grains: amaranth, buckwheat, oats, quinoa, rye, wheat.

Herbs and spices: cardamom, cinnamon, coriander, cumin, mint, mustard seeds (and greens), rosemary, sage, thyme, turmeric.

> Some of the world's tastiest cheeses are made from sheep or goat's milk. Try Roquefort, feta, manchego, ricotta and some great English ones too – have fun searching for them

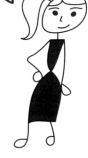

> 'Rich, fatty foods are like destiny: they too, shape our ends.'
>
> ANON

Meat

Meat is not the only protein! For some people, that comes as a revelation: we're conditioned from an early age to believe that meat is the best way to get the protein we need to help us stay strong, repair our bodies and build hair, nails, muscles, ligaments and skin.

To find out how much protein you need to eat each day, multiply your body weight in kg by 0.8g. For example, a 60kg woman will need 60 x 0.8g = 48g protein per day. If you exercise often, are pregnant, lactating or elderly, you will need more than this.

But nobody tells us that the protein in meat and poultry comes at a very high cost. It triggers all five of the ageing body processes; it's loaded with saturated fats without containing any protective antioxidants and phytonutrients; and it is hugely calorific – a 2010 study shows that for every 250g meat eaten daily, a person gains 2kg over a 5-year period.

There are **many delicious youthing alternatives to meat** – just try out some of the healthy proteins listed on page 89. If you want a leaner, more youthful body, eat meat (and make sure it's the right kind – see opposite) only once a week.

SEVEN REASONS TO CUT BACK ON MEAT

1 It is one of the most acid-forming foodstuffs. As we age, the kidneys become less effective at eliminating excess acid so calcium (an alkaline) is pulled from bones, skin, teeth, hair and nails to buffer it. Studies show that women on diets high in meat have over three times the rate of bone loss and fracture than those who get most of their protein from plant sources.

2 It causes chronic inflammation: red meats (especially beef and pork) contain high levels of saturated fats, a sugar molecule

(Neu5Gc) and a fatty acid called arachidonic acid, all of which provoke inflammation.

3 Processed meats such as hamburgers, sausages and hot dogs are also high in inflammatory, cancer-causing sulphites and nitrites. One study shows that eating 50g of processed meat a day (that's one sausage) raises your cancer risk by a fifth.

4 It irritates the gut: increased protein intake from a high-meat diet causes toxic build up in the digestive system by metabolizing into ammonia, sulphides, indoles and other toxins linked with colitis and digestive irritation. This creates nutrient deficiencies, lowered immunity, constipation, diarrhoea and a whole spin-off of ageing symptoms.

5 It may cause hormonal imbalances: the fat in red meat has been found to raise insulin levels, which increases the risk of diabetes.

6 Frying, grilling and barbecuing meat also creates dangerous DNA altering, cancer-causing compounds. One 2005 study shows that regularly eating chargrilled meats doubles the incidence of pancreatic cancer.

7 It can cause oxidative stress: red meat contains high levels of absorbable iron, and overconsumption creates excess iron in the blood. This can react to produce free radicals, which cause loss of skin tone, lethargy, stiffness, low immunity, headaches, lack of concentration and clogging of the arteries.

✳ ✳ ✳

AGEING EFFECTS OF MEAT

★ Decrease in bone strength/osteoporosis
★ Early skin wrinkling
★ Heavy, sluggish feeling
★ Increased risk of cancer and other degenerative diseases
★ Joint stiffness and pain
★ Kidney stress
★ Muscle loss
★ Red, angry spots
★ Ruddy, thick skin
★ Weakened hair, nails and teeth
★ Weight gain

✳ ✳ ✳

Avoid eating these meats 100% of the time: beef and pork; sausages, bacon, ham, hamburgers and hot dogs; minced meat and barbecued, grilled and roasted meats.

EAT FISH

Fish is a good source of protein but polluted seas/rivers mean there are safety issues around the levels of mercury and other toxins it contains. **Avoid large fish** (such as tuna, marlin and swordfish), and look out for smaller fish (herring, mackerel, salmon, sardines, trout) carrying the blue and white logo of the Marine Stewardship Council, which means they are *sustainably fished.*

See page 89 for other foods that are rich in youthing proteins.

'As for butter versus margarine,
I trust cows more than chemists,'

JOAN GUSSOW, NUTRITIONIST

'Bad' fats

Everyone is confused about fats – what kinds we should eat, what kinds we should avoid. Fats are vital for effective youthing: they maintain cell structure, help the body absorb the fat-soluble vitamins A, D, E and K, boost immunity, give you healthy looking skin, help your brain work, lift mood and provide energy. Yet some fats are intrinsically bad for you (trans-fats) and others can cause ageing free-radical damage in the body if they're stored wrongly or heated to high temperatures (polyunsaturates). This leaves us with the only safe health-giving fat in liquid form, the monounsaturated fat. Fats are also high in calories – twice as high as protein or carbohydrates!

TURN TO WHOLE FOODS

When we think of 'fats' we tend to think of the stuff we cook or spread with – butter, margarine, oils. Yet fats are in most foods we eat, including meat, fish, dairy, grains, nuts, seeds – even fruit and vegetables. For youthing purposes, it's ideal to get **most of your fats from whole foods** – from almonds rather than almond oil, from sunflower seeds rather than sunflower oil. Why? Because even healthy nut and seed oils are refined at high temperatures, which not only denature them but make them *harder for the body to process.* That said, we do need fats and oils for cooking and taste – and also to supply the two essential fatty acids that our bodies cannot produce, alpha-linolenic acid (ALA) and linoleic acid (LA).

To look and feel at your best, there is one simple fat rule: avoid 'bad' processed fats and eat 'good' fats, in the right quantities. That means decreasing your intake of trans-fats/hydrogenated fats (margarines, deep-fat cooking oils, the fats in processed foods), saturated fats from animal sources (butter, cheese and red meat) and even so-called healthy polyunsaturates (sunflower, safflower oil), which are unstable at high temperatures. Instead, **eat monounsaturated fats such as olive and rapeseed oil,** and try to eat more omega-3 fatty acids and less omega-6 fatty acids – for more on that, see overleaf.

WHAT MAKES A FAT 'GOOD' OR 'BAD'?

Every cell in our body has a protective outer covering made up of protein and fats, and the fats you eat affect its 'fluidity'. The typical western diet is high in 'bad' fats (especially trans-fats and animal-based saturated fats), which cause cell membranes to become less fluid, losing their ability to hold nutrients and water and process chemical messages. It's thought this **lack of fluidity is the trigger for many ageing symptoms** including decline in skin quality, inflammation, allergies, acne, depression, PMT, joint pain and osteoarthritis.

AVOID TRANS-FATS

Trans-fats – otherwise known as hydrogenated or partially hydrogenated fats – are chemically produced fats that are solid or semi-solid at room temperatures. They include margarines, lard (shortening) and deep-fat cooking oils. These fats are difficult for the body to process and are *supreme anti-youthers:*

★ They cause four of the ageing processes – inflammation, acidification, oxidation and hormonal imbalance. The body cannot process the Z-shaped molecules in trans-fats so they accumulate, interfering with cell functioning. Trans-fats have been banned in Denmark and manufacturers in Britain are voluntarily phasing them out, but they are still widely used in processed foods including biscuits, cakes, pies, crisps, ice creams, fast foods, cream substitutes and oils for deep-frying.

★ They make you depressed: since 1945, depression has become 20 times more prevalent in developed countries. The brain contains more lipids (fats) than any other body organ, and researchers believe that changes in our intake of dietary fat – we now eat more

AGEING EFFECTS OF 'BAD' FATS
★ Allergies
★ Breast pain and PMT
★ Cravings for high-fat foods
★ Difficult menopause
★ Feelings of anger and aggression
★ Gas, diarrhoea, constipation, as trans-fats are not well digested
★ High blood pressure
★ Inflammation
★ Inflammatory digestive problems, such as colitis and IBS
★ Lack of energy
★ Low mood
★ Osteoarthritis
★ Skin conditions, such as acne
★ Sleeping difficulties

THE BENEFITS OF GOOD FATS

When you eat the right kind and right amount of good fats your absorption of fat-soluble vitamins improves and you'll notice:

★ Better, clearer skin
★ Faster wound healing
★ Improved concentration and performance
★ Improved digestion
★ Improved sleep
★ Increased energy
★ Less inflammation
★ Lighter mood
★ More stamina
★ Reduced sugar/carb cravings

high-fat processed foods, refined and trans-fats – may have played a part in this rise. Spanish research recently found that eating high levels of trans-fats makes you 48% more likely to become depressed.

★ They are worse for heart health than saturated fats. Trans-fats clog the arteries and increase the risk of coronary heart disease. While both saturated and trans-fats raise the level of bad (LDL) cholesterol in the blood, trans-fats also lower the levels of good (HDL) cholesterol, increasing the risk of degenerative diseases.

★ They may lead to blood sugar disorders: trans-fats disrupt the action of insulin. Eating a diet that is higher in monounsaturates instead (olive oil, rapeseed oil) improves your insulin sensitivity and protects you against diabetes.

FIVE FAT-BUSTING STEPS

1 Make sure that no more than 20–30% of your diet comes from fats – that's 400–600 kcal of a typical 2,000 kcal a day diet (about 45–65g fat intake per day). And that no more than 10% of this is from saturated fats.

2 Focus on eating 'natural' unprocessed fats from oily fish, olives, avocado, goat/sheep products, soya, nuts and seeds and their oils (olive oil, rapeseed oil, coconut oil and flaxseed oil are good choices). It's better to eat full-fat than processed low-fat anything, and extra-virgin cold-pressed oils rather than refined oils, which have most of the goodness taken out of them.

3 Get a 2:1 balance of omega-6 to omega-3 fats in your diet. Most of us eat 20 times more omega-6s (found in processed foods, soya, safflower and sunflower oils) than omega-3s. Cut back on omega-6s and increase your omega-3 intake by eating more oily fish (mackerel, herring, salmon and sardines), making salad dressings from flaxseed oil, and nibbling on walnuts and hemp seeds. This will also ensure you get all the essential fatty acids (LAs and ALAs) you need.

4 Avoid any foods with the phrases 'hydrogenated' or 'partially hydrogenated' on their labels as this indicates the presence of trans-fats.

5 Don't eat deep-fried anything, especially in a restaurant or fast food outlet. Deep-frying is often done in trans-fats, as they are cheap, have a long shelf life and can be reused many times.

COOKING OILS

When cooking, choose oils that **remain stable when they are heated.** Unstable polyunsaturates (corn, safflower, soya, sunflower and generic 'vegetable' oils) tend to break down and become toxic at higher temperatures, so avoid cooking with them. Instead use coconut oil, which is stable at high temperatures, or oils that contain mostly monounsaturated fats – avocado, macadamia nut, olive and rapeseed oils. When baking, use goat's butter (you can grease tins with this too).

BUYING AND STORING OILS

Fats should be carefully stored. Polyunsaturates are unstable and break down to produce anti-youthing free radicals when they are exposed to heat, light and oxygen (though they are often deodorized so you may not smell the rancidity). For best youthing, buy oils from a shop with a high turnover rate, and go for extra-virgin, cold-pressed, unrefined, organic oils wherever possible. *Store oils in a cool, dark place* and use within 6 months. Delicate omega-3 fatty acids, such as flaxseed oil, need to be protected from heat, light and oxygen: buy them in dark bottles and store in the fridge to stop oxidation.

COCONUT OIL
COCONUT OIL IS A 'SATURATED FAT' – A PHRASE THAT USUALLY MAKES ALARM BELLS RING. BUT BECAUSE IT IS PLANT BASED, IT CONTAINS SHORT AND MEDIUM-CHAIN TRIGLYCERIDES, WHICH ARE HEALTHIER FOR YOU THAN THE LONG-CHAIN TRIGLYCERIDES FOUND IN SATURATED ANIMAL FATS. THE LIVER BURNS SHORTER-CHAIN TRIGLYCERIDES AS ENERGY SO, DESPITE COCONUT OIL BEING HIGHLY CALORIFIC, IT CAN ACTUALLY HELP WITH WEIGHT LOSS – ONE 2009 STUDY SHOWS WOMEN AGED 20–40 HAVE SMALLER WAISTS AFTER EATING COCONUT OIL FOR 12 WEEKS. IT MAY LOWER BLOOD CHOLESTEROL TOO. ALL OF WHICH MAKE IT A TOP YOUTHING CHOICE.

I'm a huge fan of coconut oil as it tastes wonderful. Try it on baked potato instead of butter, or in curries, casseroles and stews.

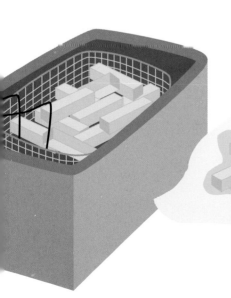

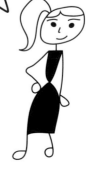

3

FIVE BEST
YOUTHING
FOODS

Do you really choose what foods you eat? Or is your diet largely a matter of habit (toast for breakfast, that latte on the way to work …), upbringing (your family always ate white bread not brown) and circumstances (office hours, eating out, family, lack of time). Well, I'd like to shake all that up. I'd like to throw 'habit' out of the window, toss 'upbringing' into the bin, and instead **focus on giving your body the healthy, nutritious foods** it needs to kick off your personal youthing journey. Great, tasty, age-busting foods that you can eat every day, however pressed you are for time.

In this chapter, I've chosen my **five top youthing foods,** one for each category: the best detoxifier/eliminator, the best anti-inflammatory, the best antioxidant, the best alkalizer and the best hormone balancer. These foods are all great at their jobs so start eating a little of them regularly. To help you along, I've explained some simple, fast, flavoursome ways to add them to your diet. They are all good detoxifiers, too, so you can easily incorporate them into your 2-week detox when you start the **EYY Programme.**

These five foods aren't the only good youthers – far from it. You'll find an **extensive list of excellent age-busting foods** and their youthing categories in the Youthing Food Chart on pages 94–9. The long-term aim is to incorporate a wide variety of these into your diet.

But the first step, right here, right now, is to change your mind-set. Forget habit, upbringing and circumstance: if you want to start looking and feeling younger, you need to start eating youthing foods. Simple. The journey starts here.

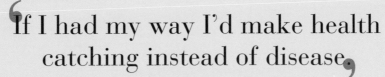

‘If I had my way I'd make health catching instead of disease’

ROBERT INGERSOLL,
19TH-CENTURY POLITICIAN

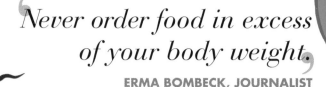

'Never order food in excess of your body weight.'

ERMA BOMBECK, JOURNALIST

Best detoxifier/eliminator: beetroot

If you're looking for a youthing food that can revitalize your whole system, this is it. Beetroot is packed with folic acid, iron, fibre, calcium, magnesium, manganese, phosphorus, potassium, carotenoids and Vitamins A, Bs and C. The rejuvenating pigments, enzyme enhancers, toxin neutralizers, immune system builders and blood pressure equalizers it contains make it your greatest friend, your daily age-defying vitamin and mineral feast. Nothing in your vegetable patch can match it.

The science behind beetroot's efficacy (see below) can seem mind-boggling, but clinical trials are conclusive. Eating beetroot will *increase your energy, stave off dementia* and, at the same time, help with the *daily detoxification* that your body desperately needs.

This little red vegetable with its earthy smell and blood red juice will cleanse your systems, oxygenate your blood and stimulate your bowels, making it the top detoxifying and eliminating vegetable around.

BEETROOT – NATURE'S THREE-WAY DETOXER

1 Beetroot's rich, purply red colour is caused by a pigment called betalain. This has a different chemical composition from the red pigments found in most other edible plants, giving it an unusual range of **detox and youthing benefits.** Betacyanin (the pigment found in red beetroot) and betaxanthin (in yellow beetroot) are highly antioxidant and anti-inflammatory, and hugely efficient at neutralizing toxins. They do this by triggering enzymes, which attach themselves to toxins, essentially changing their chemical composition so they become water-soluble and can easily be excreted from the body. This makes beetroot a good helper if you've been out for the night and had a bit too much to drink. Next morning, drinking a big glass of homemade beetroot juice (you can mix it with other veg, see pages 104–6, to make it more palatable) will help break down and eliminate the toxins from the body more quickly and get you back to feeling your best.

2 The high fibre content of beetroot is important for *immune-enhancing and detoxing.* Around 70% of the body's immune system is located in the gut and evidence shows that eating beetroot causes changes in the intestinal flora which have a positive impact on immune health – and, of course, keep the contents of the colon moving along healthily, the first step towards youthing and optimum health.

3 Beetroot is an excellent source of betaine, a liver-protecting nutrient. When the liver is functioning well, you have **higher energy levels** and **weight loss is easier to achieve.** Betaine works as a 'methyl donor', giving up methyl molecules to promote the liver's detox and fat processing functions and generating cellular renewal. Betaine also gives protection against the chemical damage caused by diabetes and alcohol.

JUICING FOR YOUTH

Beetroot juice has great rejuvenating benefits.

★ Drinking 500ml a day has been shown to **lower resting heartbeat** and **raise stamina levels.** Studies show you can then exercise for up to 16% longer before getting tired. This has real implications for anyone trying to reach youthful fitness levels: it means you can do more exercise, get fitter more quickly, and stay fit more easily. Fitness has an important effect on attitude and mood, making you feel younger, less stressed, with *more energy and enthusiasm for life.*

★ Drinking a large 500ml glass of beetroot juice significantly **lowers blood pressure** for up to 24 hours afterwards. Scientists believe

BEET GREENS contain oxalic acid, which can interfere with calcium absorption, so don't eat if you have arthritis, kidney or gall bladder problems.

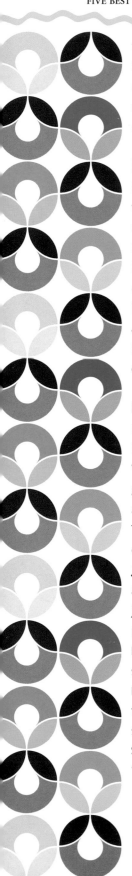

this occurs because the high level of nitrates in the juice convert in the body to nitric oxide. This relaxes blood vessels, lowers blood pressure and allows oxygen-rich blood to pump more easily around the system, creating a **healthier heart and cardiovascular system** – the engine room of youthing.

KEEPING DNA HAPPY

Beetroot is abundant in folic acid, one of the most important youthing vitamins – yet this is the world's most common vitamin deficiency. Folic acid is crucial to the body's ongoing process of cell division and DNA repair. If you don't get enough, you're likely to suffer from anaemia, diarrhoea, and be at risk of degenerative diseases. During the early stages of pregnancy, the developing foetus needs especially high levels of folic acid to prevent neural birth defects such as spina bifida. *Beetroot is a rich natural source of folic acid,* containing about 80 micrograms per 100g (RDA: 200mg for adults; 400mg for pregnant women). **For healthy, youthing cell division, eat some every day.**

EAT THE BEET

Beetroot greens (including their red stalks) have even greater nutritional benefits than the roots – they are richer in calcium, iron, carotenoids, and Vitamins A & C, and taste nicely bitter too. Add them raw into salads or gently steam as you would Swiss chard or spinach. The roots are sweeter, and delicious raw or cooked. **Aim to eat about 2 to 3 small beetroot a day.** Try red, white and yellow beetroot – they taste slightly different but are *equally as youthing.* Eat them:

Juiced: beetroot juice is a powerful detoxer, so start slowly by diluting half and half with carrot, cucumber and/or celery. After a few weeks, try beetroot juice straight up or with a shot of lemon juice to cut the sweetness (see also pages 102–7).

Raw: peeled and grated or cut into small chunks, raw beetroot adds a sharp, sweet crunch to salads.

Roasted: wash unpeeled beetroot, coat lightly in oil, place on a baking tray in the oven for 40 minutes at 190°C/Gas mark 5, or until cooked. Nudge off the skins before you eat.

Steamed: leave the root end and a bit of stem on unpeeled beetroot to stop 'bleeding'. Steam for about 15 minutes (or longer for large beetroot, but try to minimize cooking time as it can destroy beetroot's nutritional benefit). Peel before eating.

Vacuum-packed: on the supermarket shelves, it's much easier to find longlife vacuum-packed beetroot than fresh. This is precooked at high temperatures, which kills some of the nutrients, and may also have additives such as sugar, vinegar or other acid (to brighten the colour), or bicarbonate of soda or other alkali (to make them a deeper purple). Cooking your own raw fresh beetroot at home is a better youthing option and they taste sweet and nutty, not soft and mushy, much more delicious.

THE COLOUR PURPLE

Beetroot can turn urine red – a harmless condition called 'beeturia'. Your stools can also be affected, and if this happens within 12 hours of eating beetroot, your food is probably being digested too quickly. Aid your gut by taking a daily probiotic or eating goat/sheep's milk yoghurt.

> *
> *If you don't like beetroot but still want a nutrient-dense daily detox, eat watercress and cabbage to detox your liver, kidneys, lymphs and colon.*
> *

See the Youthing Food Chart on pages 94–9 for more detoxifying/eliminating foods.

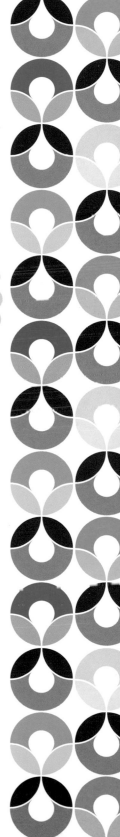

* * *

YOUTHING BENEFITS OF BEETROOT

- ★ Aids memory and decreases the risk of dementia by bringing blood to the brain
- ★ Aids weight loss, thanks to its detox properties
- ★ Detoxes the body and keeps the liver healthy
- ★ Diminishes skin-related ageing such as wrinkles and liver spots
- ★ Improves vision by increasing the oxidative supply to the retina
- ★ Increases regularity of bowel movements and the balance of intestinal flora
- ★ Increases stamina and vitality
- ★ Lowers blood pressure and blood cholesterol

* * *

'Adam and Eve ate the first vitamins, including the package,'

E.R. SQUIBB, PHARMACIST

Best anti-inflammatory: turmeric

Look in your spice cupboard – there's probably a jar of turmeric languishing there right now. Well, pull it out or, even better, go buy a new one, because this gorgeously vibrant yellow-orange spice is one of nature's most powerful anti-inflammatories, and one that I'd encourage you to start incorporating into your diet every day.

Chronic inflammation is now considered the **most important factor in early ageing** – scientists believe it encourages premature lines, loss of muscle tone, joint pain, fatigue and allergies as well as being linked to many major age-related diseases (cancer, Alzheimer's and diabetes among them). Turmeric can *help combat inflammation* in the body: it acts on a chemical level like a master switch, shutting down inflammation-causing enzymes. It's widely used in Indian and Asian cooking to soothe irritation and swelling in the body and also applied topically to inflamed skin or muscles to enhance healing – in fact Band-Aid make a turmeric plaster specially for the Indian market.

The active ingredient is curcumin, an inflammation-damping polyphenol responsible for the spice's intense orange-gold colour. There is a great deal of exciting research going on into curcumin's benefits, and results so far seem to indicate that it can combat fatigue, prevent and repair cell and tissue destruction, boost the autoimmune response (which often declines as we age), lower 'bad' LDL cholesterol and help prevent the formation of plaque, support the hormonal action of the adrenals – the body's anti-stress glands – and have a youthing

If you have arthritis, gastritis, laryngitis or anything else ending in 'itis' (which means 'inflammation'), turmeric can probably help.

effect on joints and skin. It's a great all-round rejuvenator: a vigorous antioxidant, liver protector, immune enhancer and hormone balancer, and **an effective and powerful instrument for the youthing tool box.**

TURMERIC: INFLAMMATION BUSTER!

★ Turmeric is a **potent anti-inflammatory,** as effective as anti-inflammatory drugs like ibuprofen and aspirin, and hydrocortisone (a steroid). Unlike them, it doesn't cause any unpleasant side effects such as stomach upsets, ulcers, intestinal bleeding or lowered white blood count. It offers a safe, highly effective way to lessen and help prevent inflammation throughout the body.

★ Turmeric is *especially soothing for the digestive tract.* One in five people in Britain suffers symptoms such as bloating, gas, diarrhoea, constipation and abdominal pain – all signs of intestinal inflammation. When your gut is in distress, your body doesn't absorb nutrients properly, your liver has to work harder to process fats and toxins, your immune system is under stress (as 70% of immunity starts in the gut), and as a result of this imbalance you start to age much faster. Turmeric strengthens digestion, aids in the digestion of fats and increases the liver enzymes that metabolize toxins, all of which help reduce gut inflammation and encourage daily youthing.

★ Curcumin may **revitalize your skin.** It interacts closely with collagen, the protein in the dermis, stabilizing it and increasing its viscosity. This has the effect of accelerating wound healing, reduces scarring and generally improves skin quality. It is also very good for soothing and diminishing chronic inflammatory skin conditions.

★ Curcumin helps *ease osteoarthritis.* In one 8-month study, taking 200mg curcumin a day in a compound reduced a range of osteoarthritis symptoms by half, brought down pain, and lowered anti-inflammatory drug use and accompanying intestinal problems by 63%. People reported a vastly improved quality of life, saying they generally felt more active and 'in a better mood'.

YOUTHING BENEFITS OF TURMERIC

★ Better liver detox
★ Better wound healing, less scarring
★ Boosts memory and learning capabilities
★ Cuts inflammation and pain
★ Healthier joints
★ More energy, less fatigue
★ More youthful-looking skin
★ Protects against cancers
★ Relief of stomach problems – gas, diarrhoea, colitis, indigestion
★ Sweeter mood!

THAT YOUTHING FEELING ...

★ **Turmeric seems to youth the brain!** A 2006 study shows that older people who eat turmeric occasionally or often have better functioning brains in areas of memory, concentration, language and spatial perception than those who never eat it. In lab tests, curcumin also protected against Alzheimer's disease (AD) by reducing the levels of amyloid (a tissue-destroying protein deposit found in the brain of AD sufferers) by up to 50%.

★ Curcumin can help *destress* and combat depression and anxiety too. It's one of the few things in life (intense exercise is another) that encourages the birth of new brain cells in the hippocampus, the area of the brain that shows atrophy in people with depression/anxiety.

★ Turmeric generally **helps you feel better,** by reducing the levels of Substance P – a neurotransmitter that sends pain signals from inflamed tissues to the brain. Regular doses mean fewer of the joint and muscular aches that many people experience as they grow older.

Turmeric can stain worktops, clothes and hands, so take care when using it. Dried turmeric doesn't stain as badly and provides equally potent youthing effects (provided your bottle hasn't been around for over a year).

SPICE UP YOUR DIET

Turmeric comes fresh as a rhizome (an underground stem like ginger that you can buy from Indian food shops) or you can find dried turmeric in most supermarkets. Buy organic if you can. Aim to eat 1 tsp of dried turmeric or a thumb-sized piece of fresh root, peeled and sliced, every day. Turmeric is very well tolerated by the body, even in large doses (up to 12g a day). *Arthritis sufferers* might like to take a turmeric/curcumin supplement as well as adding it to their diet. Here are some tasty ways to get turmeric into your diet:

Juice: add ¼ tsp dried turmeric to homemade fruit and veg juices.

Sprinkle: add dried turmeric over scrambled eggs, omelettes, salads ...

Soup: ½ tsp gives a delicious flavour to veg, chicken and lentil soups.

Stir-fry: start off your stir-fry with onions, oil and turmeric – the foundation of many great Indian dishes.

Salad dressing: mix ½ tsp turmeric with olive oil and lemon juice for a fast, tasty dressing.

Veg: toss cauliflower, parsnips and sweet potatoes in turmeric (mix with cinnamon, ginger and pepper to add extra flavour) before roasting.

Curry powder: make your own curry mix using fresh or dried turmeric and other curry spices, such as coriander, cumin, ginger and cayenne.

With grains: add 1 tsp turmeric to the water when you cook brown/black rice, quinoa and amaranth.

Pickled: peel fresh turmeric root and slice into fine matchsticks. Cover with lemon or lime juice, a shake of Himalayan salt and leave – it will keep in the fridge for a couple of weeks. Use as a pickle or on salads.

Paste: in a pan, simmer 25g dried turmeric with 125ml water to a thick paste. Cool. Roll into large pills with a little honey to taste, and swallow; or add 1 tsp of paste to juice or tea and drink. Will keep in fridge for 1 week.

Golden chai: see page 107.

See the Youthing Food Chart on pages 94–7 for more anti-inflammatory foods.

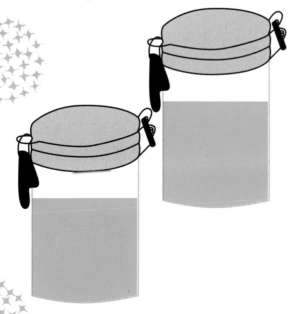

CURCUMIN AND CANCER
EXPERIMENTS HAVE SHOWN THAT CURCUMIN MAY PROTECT AGAINST CANCERS OF THE SKIN, BREAST, PROSTATE, LIVER, GUT, COLON AND STOMACH. AS A POWERFUL ANTIOXIDANT, IT MAY HELP PREVENT THE FREE-RADICAL DAMAGE THAT CAN CAUSE THE DNA MUTATIONS THAT LEAD TO CANCEROUS GROWTHS. BUT CURCUMIN ALSO SEEMS ABLE TO DESTROY CANCEROUS CELLS AND STOP THEM SPREADING. ONE STUDY SHOWS THAT AFTER 30 DAYS TAKING 1,500MG TURMERIC, HEAVY SMOKERS SHOWED A REMARKABLE DROP IN THE LEVEL OF CANCER-CAUSING COMPOUNDS IN THEIR URINE – ALMOST TO THE SAME LEVEL AS NON-SMOKERS IN THE GROUP.

'Red beans and ricely yours,'

**HOW RED BEAN FAN LOUIS ARMSTRONG
SIGNED OFF HIS LETTERS**

Best antioxidant: red beans

The red bean has several names – aduki bean, Mexican bean, small red bean, kidney bean and pinto bean – which makes navigating your way through bean land somewhat confusing. But these red-skinned beans all have one thing in common: they're packed with antioxidants. When researchers at the US Department of Agriculture analyzed the antioxidant properties of various staple foods, they found that three types of bean – small red beans, kidney beans and pinto beans – were in the top five foods, and that small red beans contained twice as many antioxidants as wild blueberries, a highly regarded 'superfood' also in the top five. Put simply, red beans are antioxidant powerhouses and for optimum youthing, can become one of your most valuable helpers.

*
Our bodies are constantly under attack from free radicals and around 10 billion molecules of the 'superoxide' radical (oxygen with an unpaired electron) bombard our cells every day. Antioxidants help to neutralize free radicals and minimize the ageing damage they cause.
*

The intensely coloured skins of red beans contain the flavonoids quercetin, tannins and anthocyanins. In tests, these compounds have been shown to *pack a bigger antioxidative punch* than many other antioxidants, protecting against cell damage – one study also showed flavonoids had a more powerful repair effect on damaged DNA than vitamin C. They can **reduce inflammation and eliminative slowdown** (two more of the ageing processes you want to minimize) and are anti-allergenic and anti-cancer.

Of course, beans are also rich in calcium, copper, iron, magnesium, manganese, phosphorus, zinc and a wide range of B vitamins as well as being a great source of fibre and low-fat protein too. So *embrace the bean* – your body will love you for it.

BEAN FEASTS

To up your antioxidant levels, aim to eat red beans regularly. This doesn't mean you have to wolf down a bean casserole every day (though four bean-containing meals a week would be very youthing!). *Beans are hugely versatile:* you can sprout them (see page 100) for salads and stir-fries and make them into soups, pastes and tea. In Japan and China, the sweet nutty taste of Sweet Aduki Bean Paste (see page 146) is much used in puddings and cakes – much healthier than our western desserts. Try these beany ideas, too:

YOUTHING BENEFITS OF RED BEANS

★ Better gut function
★ Better skin quality and elasticity
★ Help build and maintain muscle tone
★ Higher energy levels
★ Improved fertility
★ Strong, healthy teeth
★ Lower blood pressure
★ Lower cholesterol
★ Lower oestrogen levels, which may help prevent breast cancer
★ Weight loss

Bean paste: delicious spread on toast. Cook, then mash or food process with flavourings – you can make it savoury by adding liquid amino acids (from health food shops), garlic and lemon, avocado and apple cider vinegar, seaweed or miso.

Bean soups: add soaked beans to soups (add extra water as you go), simmer on low heat for an hour or more until cooked.

Tea: after simmering soaked beans for 50–60 minutes, strain off the bean water, which should be a dark reddish brown, and drink warm. If you add a bit of Japanese kombu – edible seaweed – during cooking, you'll get Japanese kombuchu bean tea, very good for detox.

Try the Beanie Brownie recipe (see page 133): it's delicious and chocolatey and no one ever realizes it contains red beans!

Sprouting: see page 100.

For other bean recipes, see pages 108–47.

BEANS 'N' GAS

If your heart is not lifting at the thought of adding beans to your diet, it may be because you are worried about becoming socially unfriendly because of the gas they produce.

Luckily, there is a way of cooking beans that gives maximum benefits and minimum side effects. Beans cause smelly flatulence because they contain oligosaccharides, which cannot be digested. These pass into the intestines where gut bacteria break them down – producing foul-smelling hydrogen, methane and sulphur compounds, which unfortunately have to come out somewhere.

If you eat beans from a can, you are well on the way to suffering no side effects, as the oligosaccharides are already partially broken down. But if you use dried beans, **soak them overnight,** then boil for about 1 hour (pinto beans will take longer). If you don't have that much time, add ¼ tsp bicarbonate of soda to each cup of beans, cover with water, bring to the boil and then boil for a further 2 minutes. Set the beans aside to soak for an hour. Then simmer the beans for about 45 minutes until they are ready. The bicarbonate breaks down oligosaccharides and reduces cooking time – though the

Canned red beans are much more convenient than dried, and contain most of the antioxidants and nutrients, so are good for youthing too. Look for tins that don't have added salt or sugar, and rinse beans well before you eat them.

Beans contain a moderate amount of purines, so if you have a tendency to gout or kidney stones consider limiting your intake.

beans might be slightly mushier than those left to soak overnight. Gaswise, *this method should improve things dramatically.*

BEAN EATERS ARE GENERALLY SLIMMER ROUND THE MIDDLE THAN NON-BEAN EATERS – ONE STUDY SHOWED THEY WEIGHED 3KG LESS AND HAD LESS ABDOMINAL FAT, EVEN THOUGH THEY ATE 200 KCALS A DAY MORE.

If you still find yourself suffering, add 1 tsp asafoetida (a pungent spice extracted from giant fennel used for this purpose in Indian cooking) to beans while they cook.

For extra nutritional benefits, **try sprouting your beans.** It increases their vitamin content, makes them more easily digestible (so again less gas!), and gives you a cheap, healthy, organic food on perpetual stand-by (see page 100).

See the Youthing Food Chart on pages 94–9 for more antioxidant foods.

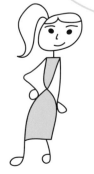

Beans give you a big plate of protein without the saturated fats, hormones or other toxic chemicals you find in meat!

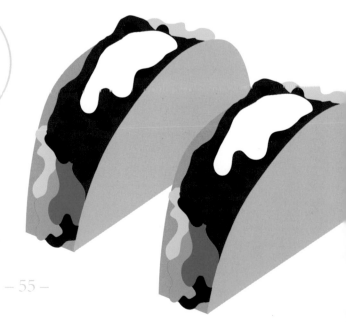

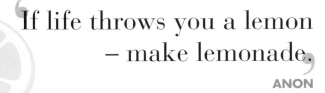

'If life throughs you a lemon
– make lemonade,'

'If life throws you a lemon
– make lemonade,

ANON

Best alkalizer: lemon

When it comes to choosing the most alkalizing food, there is no contest – the sweet-sharp kick of lemon wins hands down. This bright and beautiful fruit is a great alkalizer and, as one of nature's healthiest and most versatile all-rounders, is fantastically easy to include in your daily diet. You can add lemon juice, lemon slices or a sliver of zest to just about every dish you prepare, sweet or savoury, at breakfast, lunch and dinner – and to drinks too. It's a flavour enhancer that makes food taste better, cutting the oiliness of a salad dressing and even giving fresh fruit like pears an extra zip.

*

Give your day a powerful alkalizing start by drinking a glass of lemon juice and warm water before you do anything else. It helps the body flush away the liver's by-products. Use a straw so the acid doesn't harm tooth enamel.

*

On the tongue, lemon is acidic – it contains about 8% citric acid – but once digested it metabolizes to an alkaline state (citrate), tilting the body's intracellular fluid towards a healthy alkalinity. This is very helpful as we age, as years of bad nutrition, alcohol and lack of exercise slow the body's ability to sustain its optimum alkaline state. As explained in acifidication (see pages 20–3), an acid-forming diet can cause wrinkles, dry skin, joint stiffness, fatigue and bone loss.

EATING A DIET RICH IN ALKALIZING FOODS SUCH AS LEMONS – SUPPORTED BY OTHER FRUIT AND VEG – CAN HALT AND REVERSE THESE AGEING PROBLEMS.

Lemons are famously high in vitamin C, but they also contain vitamin A, various B vitamins, and the minerals calcium, potassium, magnesium, iron and phosphorus. Regular lemon intake stimulates the production of enzymes and digestive juices in the stomach, *enhancing the absorption of iron and calcium.* This too counteracts acidification, helping to keep bones, teeth and gums strong and improving the uptake of mood neurotransmitters such as serotonin and dopamine – essential for an **upbeat and youthful attitude to life.**

In an alkaline state, every system in the body works at its highest performance level and you'll soon notice the knock-on effects – fewer health niggles but also subtle changes to your looks, attitude and wellbeing. This is the youthing effect in action: soon skin will glow, eyes will become whiter and brighter, you'll stand tall because your joints and muscles are strong, you'll feel positive and forward-thinking – you're firing on all cylinders and will look and feel years younger.

LEMON POWER!

Lemon has many exciting youthing benefits:

★ It's high in vitamin C, which helps with **speedy skin repair** – another process that slows as we age. Vitamin C is needed to produce collagen, the vital protein that keeps skin looking young.

★ It *improves digestion* by stimulating stomach and digestive juices – minimizing bloating, heartburn, nausea, constipation and other uncomfortable digestive problems that increase with age ...

★ ... which, in turn, *helps you drop pounds.* Recent research shows that people eating a diet high in vitamin C have better digestive systems and are more likely to lose weight.

★ **Lemon can lessen sugar cravings.** Pectin, the indigestible natural fibre in lemon skin, becomes thick and gel-like in the gut, slowing down the absorption of glucose and balancing blood sugar levels. That smooths out those nasty, sugar-induced insulin spikes that make you crave sweet, high-fat foods. Indeed, one study shows that pectin makes you feel full for up to 4 hours. Adding a whole lemon to juices or a bit of peel in savoury dishes means you'll get the pectin benefits.

YOUTHING BENEFITS OF LEMONS

★ Avoid sugar cravings
★ Boost immunity
★ Healthy spot-free skin
★ Keep bones and joints healthy and strong
★ Improve detoxification
★ Improve digestion
★ Lose weight more easily
★ Lower blood pressure and bad LDL cholesterol
★ Prevent varicose veins
★ Raise your mood!
★ Stop red, broken veins appearing on your face

★ Lemon *helps prevent broken veins.* The citrus bioflavonoids it contains increase intracellular levels of vitamin C, strengthen capillaries and improve blood flow – protecting against broken veins, varicose veins and piles, boosting circulation (no more cold hands and feet!) and lowering blood pressure.

★ Lemon is **good for bones and joints.** Its high calcium content helps maintain bones; and its high levels of vitamin C promote the development of collagen-rich connective tissues, helping joints stay strong and flexible. Lemon is traditionally used to treat rheumatism and arthritis – one study shows that people with a low intake of vitamin C were over three times more likely to suffer inflammatory arthritis than those with a high intake.

★ Lemon helps *lower levels of LDL,* the 'bad' cholesterol that causes plaque deposits to build up in the arteries.

★ Lemon is an excellent detoxer, stimulating the cleansing function of the liver and pancreas, so waste products get quickly flushed away, **keeping skin clear and spot-free.** Detoxing also prevents the build-up of uric acid, which is anti-youthing and causes arthritis and gout.

★ Lemon has diuretic properties, *helping the body get rid of excess water retention* and reducing swelling – which makes it a good anti-inflammatory as well.

★ Vitamin C helps boost the immune system, so **fewer colds and infections.**

BUYING LEMONS

Look for lemons that are thin-skinned yet heavy – they contain more juice – and with a fine-grained and fully yellow skin (greenish lemons are unripe, so avoid). **As always, buy organic if you can,** to avoid pesticides and other toxins. Lemons are often waxed to increase shelf life and give them a glossy shine. Some waxes such as carnauba wax and wood resins come from edible plant sources (and are sometimes used on organic fruit), others contain ethanol, milk casein, insects and petroleum-based products. If you're eating the zest and skin, make sure you buy organic and unwaxed.

No food is more versatile than a lemon. It works as an alkalizer, detoxer, beauty treatment, condiment, in juices, soups, main courses, puddings, teas ... And it's good for colds and flu too!

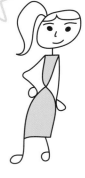

EATING LEMONS

Lemons are probably the easiest of the five foods to incorporate into your daily diet by adding a squeeze of juice or a bit of peel to your meals. Try some of these ideas:

Some people are allergic to lemon peel, and it contains oxalates, which can cause problems for those with kidney stones or gall bladder complaints.

Juices: when juicing, add a lemon (skin and all, if organic). It transforms veggie juices from the ordinary to the sublime and cuts residual sweetness from exotic fruit juices with a mango/banana/papaya base as well. If you find the juice too tart, peel the lemon and use the flesh only – the zest is the most intensely lemony bit.

Drinks: add a slice of lemon to black/green tea, herbal teas and water; make lemonade (use agave nectar instead of sugar); or concoct your own summer drink by juicing 2 lemons, 2 sprigs of mint, 2 cucumbers and then mixing with soda water to taste.

Salad dressings and sauces: lemon is a good substitute for vinegar, giving a subtler flavour.

As a condiment: mash lemon peel, garlic, parsley and a sliver of olive oil and eat with fish and meats (the Italians call this gremolata).

As a salt substitute: serve lemon wedges instead of salt at the table – great for your blood pressure.

Soups: add a slice of peel to soups.

Main courses: fish, shellfish, white meat, poultry, lentil dishes and tofu all benefit from being cooked with lemon.

With fruit: delicious squeezed over white flesh fruit, such as apples and peaches – lemon juice also stops them browning.

In breakfasts and puddings: see recipes on pages 108–10 and 131–5.

See the Youthing Food Chart on pages 94–9 for more alkalizing foods.

> 'With enough garlic, you can eat anything, even *The Sunday Times*.'
>
> JANE PHILLIMORE, JOURNALIST

Best hormone balancer: garlic

When hormones are well balanced, everything in the body works well. It's not just your sex life that improves: skin is healthy and clear; hair is shiny; the immune system, blood pressure and sugar levels are all under control; tummy fat disappears; energy, stamina and mood are high and you feel physically and mentally in tune.

> *
>
> *Garlic is great for youthing skin. In lab tests, garlic helped fibroblasts (the cells that maintain the structural integrity of skin) live longer and reproduce more healthily – which means firmer, plumper, better quality skin.*
>
> *

How to achieve this youthful state? Garlic is my first choice as an *all-round hormonal helper*. It can aid liver detox, improve digestion, lower cholesterol and blood pressure. It is antioxidant, antibacterial, antiviral and antifungal. In short, it helps balance and reboot almost every body system to give the youthing process a huge boost – even helping to minimize the symptoms of declining oestrogen or testosterone that are inevitable as we age.

> To avoid garlic breath, take it with a small glass of milk (nut, sheep, goat), chew on fennel, orange skin, or a few sprigs of parsley, basil or mint.

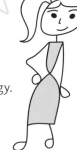

HORMONAL HIGHS

Garlic can help balance hormones in a variety of ways:

★ It contains vitamin B6, which helps with serotonin production and also corrects high cortisol levels – a cause of frequent night waking. Lower cortisol means you'll **fight stress better, sleep better** (very youthing) and increase energy.

★ The sulphides in garlic have been shown to increase adrenaline and noradrenaline. These fight or flight hormones draw on fat reserves for energy during stressful situations, rather than depleting muscle, like cortisol. Research is ongoing but it is suggested that eating garlic may make it **easier to lose fat and build muscle.**

★ Garlic is a top ten source of natural phytoestrogens, according to Canadian researchers who tested 121 common foods. Phytoestrogens mimic the action of oestrogen in the body, which can help peri- and post-menopausal women protect themselves against weight gain, hot flushes, mood swings, broken sleep and poor concentration and memory. It also helps calcium absorption in the gut, *keeping bones strong.*

★ The allicin in garlic combines with vitamin B1 (thiamine) to stimulate the pancreas to release insulin, which can **help regulate blood sugar levels,** stop food cravings and protect against insulin-deficient diabetes.

★ Garlic boosts **testosterone levels in rats** – researchers are now trying to find out if the same effect occurs in humans. Both women and men produce testosterone, and too little can result in less muscle, lowered libido, lack of vitality and increased body fat.

★ Garlic generally stimulates the whole endocrine system, increasing *vitality, stamina, concentration and libido.*

YOUTHING BENEFITS OF GARLIC

★ Better digestion
★ Better skin
★ Easier muscle building
★ Faster fat loss
★ Fewer food cravings
★ Higher libido, better sex
★ Immune system booster
★ Increased stamina
★ More energy and vitality
★ Raised mood

CLOVE POWER

Fresh garlic is more therapeutic than dried: try to eat a clove a day. Crush it then leave for 10 minutes before cooking – this activates the sulphur-containing compound allicin, and gives a better youthing effect. Garlic's fine, papery skin also contains six antioxidants: roast a few unpeeled cloves with other veg or on its own and eat the skins too.

See the Youthing Food Chart on pages 94–9 for more hormone-balancing foods.

Garlic lowers blood sugar, blood pressure and cholesterol and is an anti-coagulant. If you are on medication for these or any related conditions, including diabetes, check with your GP before taking high doses.

4

CHARTING PROGRESS

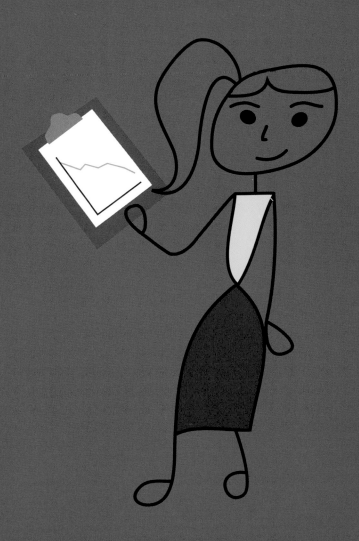

Before you start youthing, it makes sense to **find out where you're at** and what you'd **most like to change** about your body, appearance and attitudes. You also need a way to monitor progress, and keep track of improvements as time goes by. This chapter gives you the tools to do exactly that.

The detailed questionnaire on pages 64–9 will assess the **current state of your health and wellbeing**, and help you **focus on areas that need attention**. The before and after tests on pages 70–3 then **give baseline readings** in a wide variety of youthing areas: write down your answers in a notebook or diary –remember it's important to be completely honest at this stage! **Repeat the questionnaire and tests** after the 2-week **EYY Detox** and after 1 and 3 months on the **EYY Eating Plan**, as directed – it will give you an excellent indication of how much more youthful and energetic you're feeling (we quickly forget unpleasant symptoms and how debilitating they are) and how much progress you have made. Remember that progress can be measured in other, more subtle ways: it's also about self-awareness, positivity and empowering yourself to do things in a more self-controlled, productive manner. Only you can measure these changes and the sheer achievement of moving forward in difficult areas of your life.

If you follow the **EYY Programme** carefully, you'll soon notice **dramatic changes in your physique and energy levels**, which will reinforce your determination to stick to the youthing programme.

Good luck with the new you!

"Whether you think you can or whether you think you can't, you're right"

HENRY FORD, FOUNDER OF THE FORD MOTOR COMPANY

Understand your body

Before you start the **EYY Detox** or the **EYY Eating Plan**, fill in the chart below. Recording all your niggles, symptoms, irritations and ailments makes it easy to see where your body is under stress. You'll probably tick at least 10 and possibly 20 or more symptoms. Don't worry if you mark a lot of boxes: this is not a diagnosis and these symptoms may not in themselves be causing you huge problems. However, joined together they indicate that at some level, your body is not coping with the stresses and loads it is under. Notice if symptoms cluster around one body part or function, such as elimination. This indicates a problem area you need to focus on improving (read Chapter 1 for more information). Most symptoms quickly disappear once you start eating more nutritionally helpful foods.

MY SYMPTOMS CHART

Place a tick alongside any symptoms you are currently experiencing.

GUT/IMMUNITY (elimination, inflammation)					
SYMPTOM	BEFORE DETOX	AFTER DETOX	AFTER 1 MONTH	AFTER 3 MONTHS	AFTER 1 YEAR
I suffer from: ★ heartburn/acid reflux					
★ gas					
★ bloating					
★ indigestion					
★ abdominal pain					
★ low appetite					
★ overeating					
★ food cravings					
★ IBS/colitis					
★ headaches/migraine					
My stool is: ★ often runny/diarrhoea					
★ often constipated					
★ constipation/diarrhoea alternating					
I feel nauseous after eating fatty foods					
I have sugar/chocolate/alcohol cravings					
I have food sensitivities or allergies					
I have bad breath					

SYMPTOM	BEFORE DETOX	AFTER DETOX	AFTER 1 MONTH	AFTER 3 MONTHS	AFTER 1 YEAR
I regularly have:					
★ colds/flu					
★ ear, nose or throat infections					
I sneeze too often					
My nose runs after eating certain foods					
I suffer from asthma					

SKIN & NAILS (oxidation, acidification, hormonal)					
SYMPTOM	**BEFORE DETOX**	**AFTER DETOX**	**AFTER 1 MONTH**	**AFTER 3 MONTHS**	**AFTER 1 YEAR**
My skin is:					
★ dry					
★ rough					
★ oily/combination					
★ red/inflamed					
★ pale					
★ very thin					
★ prematurely lined					
★ withered/dehydrated					
★ itchy					
I have:					
★ stretch marks					
★ cellulite					
★ psoriasis/eczema					
★ acne/spots					
My palms are sweaty/clammy					
I get rashes/hives					
My heels are cracked					
My feet have corns/callouses					
My palms and feet are yellow					
I flush easily					
I bruise easily					
Cuts take a long time to heal					
My nails are:					
★ brittle					
★ thick and ridged					
★ split					
★ clubbed					
★ bluish/grey in colour					

EYES & MOUTH (oxidation, acidification, elimination)					
SYMPTOM	BEFORE DETOX	AFTER DETOX	AFTER 1 MONTH	AFTER 3 MONTHS	AFTER 1 YEAR
My eyes are: ★ bloodshot					
★ with yellow whites					
★ itchy					
★ crusty in the morning					
★ watery					
★ dry					
★ sore					
★ small and pinched-looking					
★ swollen					
I have heavy or dark bags under my eyes					
I have floaters or spots in my vision that move					
My tongue: ★ has a thick yellow/orange/white curdy coating at the back					
★ feels irritated in the morning					
★ is bright red with no coating					
★ is swollen and flabby, I can see indented teeth marks on the sides					
★ has deep cracks					
I have mouth sores/ulcers					
I have a metallic taste in the morning					
I have sore/bleeding gums					
I have gingivitis					
I have periodontal disease					
My hair is: ★ greasy, dry					
★ lifeless					
★ greying prematurely					
★ falling out					
I have dandruff					
I have a dry, itchy scalp					
WEIGHT (acidification, elimination, hormonal)					
SYMPTOM	BEFORE DETOX	AFTER DETOX	AFTER 1 MONTH	AFTER 3 MONTHS	AFTER 1 YEAR
I'm overweight					
I'm underweight					

SYMPTOM	BEFORE DETOX	AFTER DETOX	AFTER 1 MONTH	AFTER 3 MONTHS	AFTER 1 YEAR
I find it hard to lose weight					
My excess weight is all around my middle					
My muscle tone is poor					
My stamina is low					
I feel low in energy					
I don't want to exercise					

JOINTS & MUSCLES (inflammation, acidification)

SYMPTOM	BEFORE DETOX	AFTER DETOX	AFTER 1 MONTH	AFTER 3 MONTHS	AFTER 1 YEAR
One or more of my joints is painful					
My muscles often feel sore					
The knuckles in my fingers ache					
My fingers are often swollen					
My joints: ★ crack or pop ★ are stiff or painful on waking ★ are stiff or painful at night					
I have bone thinning/osteoporosis					

URINARY (acidification, hormonal)

SYMPTOM	BEFORE DETOX	AFTER DETOX	AFTER 1 MONTH	AFTER 3 MONTHS	AFTER 1 YEAR
My wee is: ★ smelly ★ dark yellow or brown ★ hot/painful					
I need to pee very frequently					
I have had cystitis/UTIs in the past month					
I often feel thirsty					
I don't sweat					
I sweat too much					

CIRCULATION (hormonal, inflammation, elimination)

SYMPTOM	BEFORE DETOX	AFTER DETOX	AFTER 1 MONTH	AFTER 3 MONTHS	AFTER 1 YEAR
My circulation is poor					
I have very white/red hands					
I can't cool down					
My feet and hands are often cold					
I feel cold all the time					
I have broken capillaries on my face/body					
I have varicose veins					
I get palpitations					
I feel breathless					

HORMONAL

SYMPTOM	BEFORE DETOX	AFTER DETOX	AFTER 1 MONTH	AFTER 3 MONTHS	AFTER 1 YEAR
I have vaginal thrush (women) or white flakes under foreskin (men)					
My periods are irregular					
I have burning feet at night					
I wake up looking puffy/ suffer from water retention					
Around my period I suffer from: ★ PMT ★ fluid retention ★ sore breasts ★ period pain					
I have the following menopausal symptoms: ★ hot flushes ★ swings ★ night sweats ★ sleep disturbances ★ weight gain ★ loss of libido ★ low energy					

MIND & EMOTIONS (all five processes)

SYMPTOM	BEFORE DETOX	AFTER DETOX	AFTER 1 MONTH	AFTER 3 MONTHS	AFTER 1 YEAR
I feel wired, I can't get to sleep at night					
I wake up during the night and can't get back to sleep					

SYMPTOM	BEFORE DETOX	AFTER DETOX	AFTER 1 MONTH	AFTER 3 MONTHS	AFTER 1 YEAR
I wake up feeling tired					
My dreams wake me up					
I fall asleep in the afternoons					
I find it hard to concentrate					
My memory is getting worse					
I often feel moody/irritable					
I feel stressed a lot of the time					
I get overwhelmed by emotion					
I fly off the handle easily					
I worry incessantly					
I am restless and agitated					
My mind is in a whirl					
I feel low/depressed					
I don't laugh much					
I feel antisocial					
I often find myself chewing my hair or nails (or other repetitive behaviour)					
I am very sensitive to alcohol					
I am more tired than normal					
I feel exhausted					
I feel old					

What youthing benefit do I want most?

_____

_____

_____

What would I most like to change about myself?

_____

_____

_____

Check your progress

The five tests below help you to monitor your progress on the **EYY Eating Plan**. If you wish, do them before you start, to give yourself a baseline reading and then as directed.

1 BODY FAT TEST

One of the best ways to monitor progress is by measuring body fat. Take regular measurements of the specific areas below and date and record them in a notebook/diary.

BODY AREA	MEASUREMENT
Upper arm	. . . .
Chest (around widest point)	. . . .
Chest, below breasts (for women)	. . . .
Waist	. . . .
Hips	. . . .
Bottom	. . . .
Upper thighs	. . . .
Above knees	. . . .
Calf	. . . .
Ankles	. . . .

If you have a problem with a particular area – say a flabby stomach or back fat – then pinch the fat there between calipers (you can buy home kits) and measure this regularly too. Body composition scales (you can buy them in department stores or online) monitor overall levels of body fat by sending a low-voltage electric current through the body. (Healthy fat ranges are around 20% to 35% for women and 10% to 25% for men, depending on age, the scale will give you a reading.) Repeat after the **EYY Detox** and then after 3 months and 6 months.

2 SKIN ELASTICITY TEST

This is a simple way to test the collagen bounce in your skin. Skin renews itself every 4–6 weeks and after a few months of youthing eating and good hydration skin can improve markedly, as the production of skin proteins collagen, elastin and keratin are boosted. Skin may start to look plumper, firmer, softer, more supple and return to normal more quickly after the test.

To take the test, relax your arm on a table, and pinch the skin on the back of your hand firmly between your thumb and forefinger for 30 seconds. Let it go, then slowly count 'one and two and three …' to see how long it takes for the skin to flatten out and for the colour to go back to normal. Compare your results to the chart below to find out the functional age of your skin. Repeat after the **EYY Detox**, then every 3 months thereafter.

WOMEN TIME	FUNCTIONAL AGE (IN YEARS)
3	under 30
4	30–40
5	40–50
6	50–60
7	60–70
8	70–80

MEN TIME	FUNCTIONAL AGE (IN YEARS)
2	under 30
3	30 40
4	40–50
5	50–60
6	60–70
7	70–80

* * *

LOVE YOUR QUIRKS

Although your physique can change, some physical features never will. For example, your proportions won't alter greatly – if you have a relatively large bum or boobs, they will remain that way compared to the rest of your body. Likewise your knobbly feet, wonky nose, chubby cheeks or other pet hates are not miraculously going to disappear. Try to positively embrace these quirks. It is youthing to accept the way you look, to feel at home in your skin. Help the process by reciting daily mantras along the lines of: 'Yes, I love my bottom, it may be large but it suits my body and is firm, sexy and cellulite-free …'

* * *

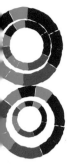

3 THE GRIN AND BARE IT TEST

Take a photograph of yourself naked or in a bikini/swimming trunks, from the front, back and side. This will feel embarrassing but grin and bear it: these pictures will be a great motivator, giving clear, dispassionate evidence of your body shape and problem areas before you start and inspiring you stick to your youthing programme.

After 3 months on the **EYY Eating Plan**, take another set of images and compare them. After this sustained period of youthing nutrition you'll notice how your body has changed: fat stores start to diminish, midriff rolls will disappear as blood sugar settles down, skin elasticity and muscle tone improve to give better definition and re-sculpt your physique. By then it will be difficult to remember what you looked like before you started youthing, so these images provide a genuine and important record of your progress. Repeat after 6 months and a year.

4 MEMORY TEST

Forgetfulness is a natural part of ageing – or is it? We've all met supersharp 70-somethings who have the thinking skills and memory power of someone 40 years younger. Memory is often more about focus and paying attention – skills available at any age. But interestingly, diet has been found to affect brain health and function and the omega-3 rich fatty acids you eat on the **EYY Eating Plan** are thought to support synaptic connections and have a positive impact on memory and cognitive function. Do the following two tests and record your results in your diary. Repeat after 3 months.

Test 1: *for visual memory*

Stare for 15 seconds at a photograph in a newspaper: one
recording a memorable event. Try to remember ten specific points about it,
then turn the newspaper over and write them down. Look at the
picture again, and mark how many points you scored.

Test 2: *for verbal memory*

Ask a friend/partner to think of ten unrelated nouns and
say them slowly out loud while you listen and try to remember them.
Wait for 2 minutes, then repeat the nouns back to your friend.
Mark down how many you scored.

5 THE FOOD ZERO TEST

We're often attracted to the foods that cause our constitutions most aggravation. The food you crave – the thing you would find hardest to give up and has become an emotional support for you (typically coffee, carbs, high-fat foods, citrus fruit, sugar, alcohol) – is normally the thing you should cut out at once, even if it is considered 'healthy', as you may be intolerant or even allergic to it. The following questions can help you identify which foods should be given zero tolerance.

To take the test, answer the questions below. If a food pops up in the answer to every question, stop eating it for a couple of weeks. If symptoms disappear, you know that specific food is the cause, so cut it out of your diet for 3 months. You can reintroduce it after this time – but monitor symptoms and if you notice any physical/emotional changes in your health and wellbeing, you know your body is intolerant of it and you should cut it out of your diet completely.

1 Which foods/drinks do you eat every day without fail?
2 Of these foods/drinks which do you feel deprived of in a day if you are unable to consume them?
3 Do you ever crave this particular food/drink so much that it distracts you?
4 Have you eaten/drunk this particular item for more than a 6-month period with no break?
5 Does this food/drink change your mood when you have it, or if it is taken from you?
6 Can you feel your body responding to the food/drink when you eat/drink it, either negatively or positively?

* * *

WAKE-UP CALL

Look back at old photographs of yourself, 5, 10, 15 or more years ago. What do you see? I bet you think: wow, I didn't look bad at all. Then remember what was going through your head at that time. Chances are you thought you were fat, or had wobbly upper arms, or a few wrinkles that you thought made you look old. But in reality you didn't look fat or old, you looked fabulous – you just couldn't see it. Recognizing this mismatch between inner and outer perception is an important wake-up call: how we think we look bears little relation to how we actually look. All that time you could have been enjoying you were beating yourself up imagining your ageing flaws. So don't waste your energy – enjoy the moment of being the age you are, wherever that is.

* * *

5

THE EYY
DETOX

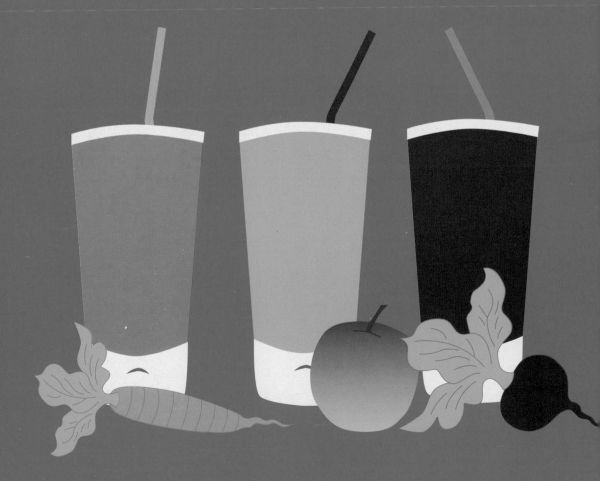

If you want to look and feel different fast, a detox is the best beginning you can give yourself. After just 2 weeks, you will **feel fresh, clean, awake, vibrant, youthful and ready for action.** A good detox changes you physically and emotionally, flushing out accumulated wastes to help liver function, and increasing enzyme production and nutrient absorption. It's a **hugely important start to youthing** as it minimizes **all five ageing processes:** it helps even out blood sugar levels and rebalance hormones, reduce inflammation, boost alkalinity, improve digestion, and increase the levels of antioxidants in the body. It also helps stop cravings and creates a healthy discipline around eating. In short, **it bounces you back from deficiency to strength,** ready to start the **EYY Eating Plan** that will nourish and sustain your youthing for life.

Detoxing is strenuous and **not advised for everyone.** If you have heart problems, are diabetic, obese, elderly, pregnant, breastfeeding, under 16, have recently had a medical operation or are recuperating from illness, are on medication including for depression/anxiety or epilepsy, this detox is not for you. If you are on the Pill, HRT or statins, please check with your GP or health professional before starting.

'Eating what stands on one leg (plants)
is better than eating what stands
on two legs (chicken, game)
which is better than eating what stands
on four legs (cows, pigs …)'
CHINESE PROVERB

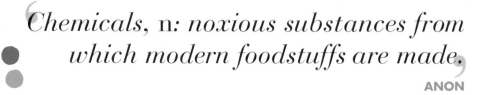

'Chemicals, n: noxious substances from which modern foodstuffs are made,'

ANON

The power of the detox

We don't pay enough attention to cleaning ourselves on the inside – until the wear and tear of ageing symptoms starts to show on the outside. Then you know it's definitely time to give the body some extra help. The major player in detox is the liver, which is responsible for metabolizing foods and harmful substances: toxins like heavy metals, alcohol, pharmaceutical and recreational drugs as well as chemical additives and preservatives. The liver breaks down these toxins through multiple chemical conversions into harmless substances that are stored in the liver, and are eventually eliminated via the other detox organs – the kidneys, lungs, lymph, digestion and skin.

When we're young and every organ is in peak condition, the body's natural toxin removal system works seamlessly. But as we age we're exposed to an accumulation of toxins. These include the thousands of unnecessary substances added to processed and junk foods – preservatives, stabilizers, artificial colourings and flavourings – plus the pesticides, fertilizers, sprout inhibitors, hormones and antibiotics used to grow plant foods and the animals we eat. But other factors play a part too:

★ Unhealthy living from stress, overwork, smoking, alcohol, prescription or recreational drugs load extra toxins into our bodies.
★ Toxins from the environment – pollution from cars, planes, industry, house paint, hair dyes, plastics, cleaning materials, new carpets – impact us on a daily basis.

The rubbish flow builds up and our bodies struggle to process these **damaging wastes.** We start to see anti-youthing signs: skin problems, fine lines, fatigue, aches and pains, indigestion, sluggish metabolism, weight gain, cellulite and memory loss.

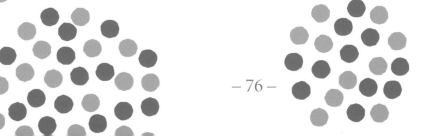

THE BEST HELP YOU CAN GIVE YOUR BODY IS TO LIGHTEN ITS LOAD.

Stop eating foods that are processed, chemically altered or full of additives. Stop drinking alcohol and caffeine. Instead, start eating healthy, additive-free foods that are packed with the phytonutrients, antioxidants and biochemical compounds the body needs to process both fat- and water-soluble toxins. Start drinking rejuvenating teas and lots of water to help the kidneys flush out accumulated wastes. Accelerate the process with herbal helpers (see page 81), which support the liver, kidneys, lymph and digestion.

To kick off the **EYY Programme,** detox for 2 weeks. People often get very anxious about changing their food routine. When you're a meat-and-two-veg kind of person and are confronted with a detox with no meat, fish, caffeine, cow's milk or grains you think 'EEFK! What's left to eat?' The answer is an incredible number of things – and lots of them. Being hungry is not part of this detox plan: you can eat as much as you like, just of the right things. Your primary aim is not to lose weight (though you almost certainly will if you need to), but to give your body the support it needs to get rid of its toxic log jam.

Over the next few pages you'll find lots of detox advice, plus eating plans for the **EYY Detox.** These contain a range of creative meal ideas and recipes to make your detox as tasty and varied as possible. Treat them as inspiration: a way to open your eyes about the imaginative, flavoursome meals you can create using healthy youthing foods.

This detox has one superb youthing effect – it eradicates around 70% of the ongoing symptoms, such as low energy, skin blemishes and indigestion, which make you feel tired and old. As your energy levels soar, you will lose a bit of weight and your skin will start to glow, you'll feel healthy and rejuvenated – and younger looking. Not bad in 2 weeks!

POSSIBLE SIDE EFFECTS

As you probably know, the first few days of detox can be painful. Giving up coffee and sugar, for example, can make you feel weak, sweaty and headachey. Normally these symptoms pass after 4 days, when your energy levels rise and you start to feel more youthful, dynamic and focused. Don't be concerned if at first you experience the following:

★ Bad breath
★ Body odour
★ Boredom!
★ Fatigue
★ Headaches (particularly if you are a coffee drinker)
★ Inability to concentrate
★ Intestinal gas
★ Irritability
★ Muscle aches and pains
★ Skin rashes
★ Spots (as the skin flushes through toxins)
★ Sugar cravings
★ Sweaty, shaky feeling

'Just because you're not sick,
it doesn't mean you're healthy,'

ANON

Ten steps
to successful detoxing

Love it or hate it, everyone knows they benefit from a detox. It's rare
not to end the 2 weeks with a sense of exhilaration and achievement.

1 Start the day with a homemade, nutrient-packed juice (see pages 102–7) or lemon
in warm water. Drink it on an empty stomach, then wait half an hour before eating
breakfast.

2 Eat breakfast, lunch and dinner every day, choosing from the list and recipes on
pages 82–5. Note that you are allowed to eat different foods in Week 1 and Week 2.

3 Choose seasonally produced organic fruit and veg. If that proves too expensive,
invest in a fruit and vegetable wash (from health food shops), which removes surface
chemicals and waxes.

4 Make sure you have some of these must-have detoxing veg in your meal or juice
every day: asparagus, beetroot, broccoli, Brussels sprouts, cabbage, cauliflower,
chard, chicory, fennel, garlic, kale, leeks, mustard seeds, onions, radish, rocket,
seaweed, sweet potato and watercress. Also raw carrots, spinach and tomatoes:
they are high in glutathione, a protein that 'escorts' toxins out of the body.

5 Make sure you eat some of these cleansing fruits every day: apples, grapefruit
(both high in glutathione), lemon, papaya and pineapple are good digestives,
supporting the detox process.

6 Make sure you get around 45g a day of protein (depending on your body weight,
see page 36) in the form of beans, chickpeas, lentils, tofu, nuts, seeds, eggs and goat/
sheep/buffalo's yoghurt/cheese. Alternate the source daily.

7 Get some omega-3 fatty acids each day: walnuts, pumpkin seeds, flaxseeds/
linseeds, kidney beans, tofu and fresh soya/edamame beans are all good sources of
omega-3s, which have anti-inflammatory properties and help with mood, immunity,
brain function and memory, firm skin and healthy nails.

8 Don't miss meals: you'll be starving by 3pm and break the detox by eating whatever is to hand. If you want a snack, have some fruit or eat your daily pudding.

9 Have a good source of still mineral or filtered water handy (see page 90) and aim to drink 8 glasses a day to flush wastes away.

10 To support the various detox organs, consider taking some of the herbal helpers on page 81.

DETOX ACCELERATORS

These will help you make faster progress during detox – and you can build them into your daily life afterwards too.

★ Get outside every day and walk about – borrow a dog if you don't have your own! Walking after eating lowers stress, strengthens muscles and reduces the amount of fats, sugars and hormones released into the bloodstream, helping the youthing process.

★ Breathe deeply: the lungs help eliminate toxins and deep breathing increases the oxygen supply to the body, which can make you feel heady and relaxed. Breathe deeply three times a day: inhale slowly to the count of four, expanding your abdomen, hold for a count of one, then slowly breathe out to a count of six. Pause and repeat five times.

★ Daily body brushing increases the detox effect by stimulating the lymph and helping release toxins through the skin. With a bristle brush, and using gentle, circular movements, start brushing the soles of your feet, move up your legs, front and back, then start at your fingers, working up your arms. Finally brush your torso front and back towards your heart. Shower afterwards.

★ Scrape your tongue every morning when you wake up (see page 156) and notice how the debris changes colour and thins during the detox. This is a sign that the body is helping to rid itself of the overload of toxins.

★ Add 6–8 drops of a soothing, sweet-smelling detox oil, such as grapefruit, fennel, geranium or ylang-ylang, to the bath to relax you and intensify the detox effect.

POSSIBLE SIDE EFFECTS

★ Better concentration
★ Clearer in the mind
★ Clear eyes
★ Feel lighter, 'cleaner'
★ Fewer sugar cravings
★ Glowing skin
★ Improved digestion
★ Less angry
★ Less anxious/panicky
★ Less foggy in the morning
★ Look and feel younger – lots of compliments!
★ More alert
★ More energy
★ No migraines/headaches
★ No PMS
★ Shinier hair
★ Sleep better
★ Wake earlier
★ Weight loss

'*I like rice. Rice is great if you're hungry and want 2,000 of something.*'

MITCH HEDBERG, COMEDIAN

Getting started

Before you start the detox, fill in the My Symptoms Chart on pages 64–9 and the tests on pages 70–3. Then complete it after the detox – and notice how many of your symptoms have disappeared ...

★ Choose 2 weeks when you don't have much on, don't have to eat out, and when you can go to bed early and get lots of rest. If this never happens, follow the tips on pages 153–5 to help you stick to your detox diet while you're out.

★ Stock your kitchen cupboard before you start: get rid of tempting foods (crisps, biscuits, chocolate, ice cream), then look at the weekly detox sheets/recipes and shop for a few days' ahead, so that you'll never be starving or low in delicious things to eat.

★ Don't think you have to cook every day – make double or even triple quantities of dishes you particularly like. Take into work for lunch or keep in the fridge/freezer.

★ The detox is not specifically about losing weight but if that is one of your aims, give yourself just one plateful of food per meal. You can pile it as high with as many vegetables as you like, but know that this is it. No more until the next meal.

If you get sugar cravings, eat a handful of nuts, fresh soya/edamame beans, raw tofu, beetroot or liquorice.

★ Carry a pen and pad around and jot down reactions or feelings that seem unusual: detox affects the mind and emotions as well as the body.

★ For the first 4 days, eat with chopsticks only. It's important because it makes you take smaller mouthfuls and eat more slowly, which aids digestion. You can buy EYY chopsticks from www.epjhealth.com.

★ Find a detox buddy: their support can make it easier if times get tough.

★ Chew to the clock: time each mouthful so you take 20 seconds to chew 'soft' food and 40 seconds for 'hard' food. This makes you more aware of what you're eating, you'll digest food better and feel less hungry. Download my Eat to the Beat chewing app from www.epjhealth.com.

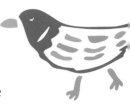

FORBIDDEN FOODS!

During detox, you should cut out:

Processed foods and ready meals, or any foods with preservatives, additives, or 'fresh' foods with a sell-by date of over a month.

Meat and fish: one interesting effect of detox is that you'll start thinking more creatively about proteins such as nuts, beans and seeds.

All cow's milk dairy products including milk, butter, cheese, cream, cottage cheese and yoghurt. (You are allowed 2 tbsp goat/sheep/buffalo's milk products a day.)

All grains in Week 1, though you reintroduce them in Week 2.

Sugar, artificial sweeteners, honey, agave nectar, maple and other syrups.

Caffeine, tea, cocoa, alcohol, fizzy or sweetened drinks.

Oils: trans-fats, margarines and polyunsaturated oils such as sunflower and safflower. Use unrefined olive, rapeseed, sesame and coconut oil instead.

Salt and anything that has salt added to it (including Himalayan salt, mineral salt and liquid aminos) unless you have low blood pressure, in which case use the good salts advised on page 33. If you want something salty, add seaweed to a dish.

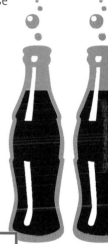

* * *

HERBAL HELPERS

Supporting your major detox organs (liver, kidneys, lymph, bowels) with herbal supplements during the detox process may help them process harmful substances, speed up recovery from side effects and enhance the eliminative effects. See www.epjhealth.com for more information.

★ For the kidneys, try aloe vera, gravel root, juniper berries, uva ursi and barley water (cook 50g pot barley with 500ml water and grated ginger, simmer until soft, strain).

★ For the liver, try milk thistle, dandelion, turmeric, yellow dock, burdock, aloe vera or chlorophyll (as chlorella, blue/green algae, kelp or spirulina) either as single or combination tinctures or teas.

★ Support your bowels with a daily dose of soothing clay and slippery elm powder, psyllium husks, flaxseeds or aloe vera.

★ For excessive bloating, chew on fennel seeds, drink ginger juice with a touch of apple (to make it palatable) or take a peppermint pearl (from chemists) after a meal.

* * *

The EYY Detox: Week 1

The first week is always a challenge. Your food choices are significantly reduced – no meat, fish, cow's dairy, grains, salt, caffeine or alcohol.

Instead you'll eat only vegetables, vegetable proteins, fruits, fats in the form of vegetable oil and one portion of dairy (2 tbsp) in the form of goat/sheep/buffalo's cheese and yoghurt. You can also eat 2 eggs a week. Eat a breakfast, light meal and main meal every day, and add pudding if you feel like something sweet.

JUICES

Start every day with a 300ml glass of one of the following fresh juices. Then wait 30 minutes or so for it to digest before eating your main breakfast.

★ Green Youthing Shake (see page 105)
★ Watercress, Beetroot & Carrot Zinger (see page 104)
★ Super-charged Spring Cleaner (see page 106)
★ Apple & Carrot Detox Speeder (see page 105)
★ Go Skin Glow (see page 104)
★ Detox Root and Beetroot Burst (see page 104)
★ Potato Juice (see page 105)

> Remember to drink your juice every day!

BREAKFAST

You can eat a hot breakfast or fruit with some goat/sheep/buffalo's yoghurt. The puddings (see opposite) can be eaten as breakfasts too.

★ Fruit salad with nuts or seeds and yoghurt
★ Fruity almond broth: 1 apple, 1 pear, handful raisins, pinch nutmeg and cinnamon simmered in 400ml Almond Milk (see page 147) until soft
★ Baked cooking apple stuffed with raisins, ginger, cinnamon, topped with crushed walnuts and yoghurt
★ Mashed banana, pinch cinnamon and nutmeg, topped with pecan nuts, Brazil nuts and yoghurt
★ Boiled or poached egg with raw veg soldiers (carrot, tomato, etc.)
★ Scrambled tofu with shiitake mushrooms, spring onions, green peppers and turmeric
★ Alkalizing herbal broth (handful of spinach, lettuce, Swiss chard, leeks, chervil, 1 litre water, blend and simmer for 20 minutes)

LIGHT MEAL

If you have lunch at work, take in a flask of one of the following youthing soups or make up one of these delicious, vitamin–packed salads.

★ Alkalizing Cannellini Bean Soup (see page 113)
★ Youthing Butternut Squash & Ginger Soup (see page 114)
★ Creamy Beetroot Detox Soup (see page 112)
★ Green Gazpacho (see page 111)
★ Antioxidant-rich Potato Salad (see page 115)
★ Spiced-up Beanie Salad (see page 116)
★ Energizing Fennel & Artichoke Salad (see page 115)

MAIN MEAL

Eat at lunch or dinner. In the evening try to eat before 7.30pm so food is properly digested and you get a better night's sleep.

★ Asian Crunchy Stir-fry (see page 130)
★ Super Youthing Stroganoff (see page 122)
★ Vitality Black Bean Curry (no rice) (see page 119)
★ Rejuvenating Lentil Detoxer (see page 129)
★ Trad Thai Curry, but without the barley (no grains) (see page 120)
★ Goat's Cheese, Aubergine & Butter Bean Bake (see page 118)
★ Soothing Coconut Dhal (see page 128)

PUDDINGS

You can eat one pudding a day, preferably at lunch (or as a snack) rather than dinner to minimize the amount of sugars you have after 7.30pm. All these puds can be eaten for breakfast, too, with some goat/sheep/buffalo's milk yoghurt.

★ Stewed apple and pear, with chopped dates, squeeze of orange juice
★ Sliced papaya with passion fruit pulp and squeeze of lime juice
★ Frozen banana: peel and freeze banana, blend, serve with blueberries
★ Blueberry Layered Coulis with a Chilli Kick (see page 132)
★ Baked banana: bake with skin on for 20 minutes (200°C),
then peel and eat with yoghurt
★ Fresh pears with orange and dried apricots

The EYY Detox: Week 2

You may add high-quality grains and breads to your diet this week, but only eat them in the morning or at lunch rather than the evening. They contain complex carbs, which make you feel full and sluggish – whereas you want to wake feeling refreshed, lean and hungy. Every day still starts with a homemade juice: a great opportunity to get your daily dose of beetroot and turmeric, as well as antioxidants, vitamins, minerals and other phytonutrients. If you don't want to cook or are short of time, continue eating vegetables and fruit, but eat a portion of vegetable protein (see page 89) every day. If you need more energy, add a portion of slow-release carbs (preferably quinoa, millet, amaranth, buckwheat and red or black rice). You can have two eggs this week.

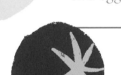

JUICES

As Week 1 (see page 82).

BREAKFAST

Add grains if desired to your breakfast – try porridge, oat groats, muesli, quinoa or rice – or continue eating the Week 1 breakfasts if you prefer something lighter.

★ Fruity porridge: cook oat groats (see page 102), quinoa, buckwheat or millet in water. Serve with nut or rice milk (see page 147), cinnamon and nutmeg, fruit (apple, banana, berries, figs) and seeds (pumpkin/sunflower)

★ Figgy Nut Bircher Muesli (see page 109) with fresh fruit

★ Youthing rice breakfast: warm up cooked brown rice in a pan with apple juice, crushed almonds, pumpkin seeds and dried cranberries

★ Two-egg omelette with toasted rye bread

★ Banana dipped in sesame seeds, sliced on to 2 slices of wheat-free toasted bread

★ Two slices of non-wheat bread with pumpkin seed spread or nut butter (see page 145)

★ Grilled tomatoes with goat's cheese and fresh tarragon

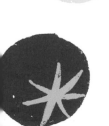
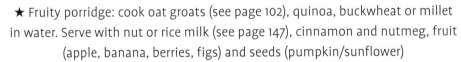

LIGHT MEAL

Eat as Week 1 or choose from the following:

★ Fennel Soup (see page 112) and Pumpkin Seed & Tomato Bread (see page 138)
★ Youth-boost Burger with Sweet Tomato Relish (see page 117)
and tomato and avocado salad
★ Super Soba Noodle Salad (see page 116)
★ Baked Beans (see page 108) on rye toast
★ Stuffed Courgettes (see page 128) with Walnut Bread (see page 139)
★ Crudités with Avocado Summer Dip (see page 137)
and Super Youthing Salsa (see page 136)
★ Steamed greens with pesto, topped with oven-baked pine nuts,
pumpkin seeds and goat's cheese

MAIN MEAL

Eat at lunch or dinner. In the evening try and eat before 7.30pm so food is properly
digested and you get a better night's sleep. Eat as Week 1 or try:

★ Roasted Root Vegetables (see page 127) and green salad
★ Antioxidant Aubergines (see page 124)
★ Youthing Coconut Curry (see page 123)
★ Borlotti Bean & Cavolo Nero Casserole (see page 125)
★ Spelt Pasta with Quick Tomato Sauce (see page 143)
★ Mushroom Barley Risotto (see page 126)
★ Sweet Beetroot Slaw with Baked Potato with Wasabi (see pages 114 and 124–5)

PUDDINGS

You can eat the same puddings as in Week 1, or try the following. Eat them
at lunch (or as a snack) rather than after dinner.

★ Fresh fruit with mashed blackberries
★ Fresh fruit with freshly squeezed orange/lime juice, and mint leaves
★ Sliced mango with lime juice and freshly grated coconut
★ Chopped dates, figs, apple, pear, almonds, walnuts with sheep's milk yoghurt
★ Creamy Coconut & Pineapple Black Rice Pud (see page 131)
★ Fruity Jelly (see page 132)
★ Vanilla Soya Custard (see page 133)

6
THE EYY EATING PLAN

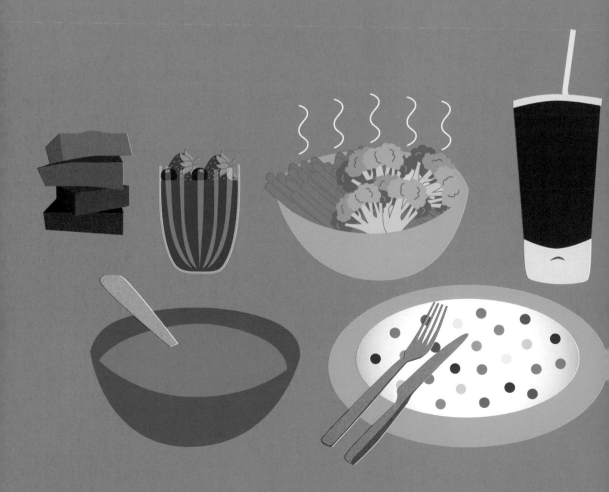

After the detox, you will be feeling rejuvenated and vibrantly alive. But now comes the hard bit – creating a healthy, youthing diet that will nourish and sustain you not just for 2 weeks but **for the rest of your life.** You want to be in peak condition every day, aware of your body and able to supply its nutritional needs. You want tasty, fabulous food that is easy to prepare and satisfying to eat. Most importantly, you want a diet that will slow down and even reverse the ageing process so you **start to look and feel younger.**

The **EYY Eating Plan** is very easy to follow. In this chapter, you'll find around 70 delicious recipes for youthing juices, breakfasts, main meals, side dishes, puddings, snacks, breads and cakes. On pages 94–9 there's a detailed **Youthing Food Chart** that tells you which foods to incorporate into your diet to counter the five malfunctions and **enhance the youthing process.** Alongside each recipe there is a colour-coded flower (see right) that highlights which youthing processes the recipe supports. Don't feel you have to follow everything precisely, **so pick and choose the ingredients** and recipes you like, and adapt them to suit your tastes. Be creative and enjoy it. It is the best youthing start to the rest of your life.

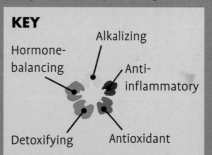

KEY
Hormone-balancing
Alkalizing
Anti-inflammatory
Detoxifying
Antioxidant

'People worry about what they eat between Christmas and New Year, but they should really worry about what they eat between New Year and Christmas'

ANON

The ten EYY Eating Plan principles

I'm against making strict rules as the **EYY Eating Plan** is about finding foods and recipes that you love and can happily eat for the rest of your life. But setting out a few principles can help you to follow the best youthing eating habits from the start.

1 Eat three regular meals a day. Skipping a meal makes you very hungry which sets off the hormone ghrelin (which creates those grinding hunger pangs in your stomach), and links with the hypothalamus to make you crave high-fat, high-calorie foods. Keeping your body fed well and regularly will minimize these cravings and help your digestive system work at its best.

2 Drink a homemade vegetable juice before breakfast every day. Leave for 30 minutes before eating breakfast. If you don't have time to make juice, squeeze half a lemon into hot water instead.

3 Eat 30% raw food every day, including your juice and fruit. Unheated foods contain more enzymes, vitamins and minerals than cooked foods. Your green juice plus a salad or side of crudités should do it.

4 Eat protein, fat and carbs at every meal. Vegetables are your most important youthing friends and should form the mainstay of your diet. Then add a little protein (see opposite), a little fat, and some unrefined carbs – the kind that comes from wholegrains and breads.

5 Regularly try different foods to get the widest range of nutrients into your body. A good guide to that is the colour of the food on your plate. So if you have a dish with salmon, pistachios and brown rice on Tuesday, have pak choi, beetroot and black beans on Wednesday.

> *Don't pig out on fruit – it is high in sugars. Limit yourself to 2–3 pieces a day. If you have a fruit salad for breakfast, that will use up your fruit quota for the day. But if you just have one kiwi fruit, you can have one or two more pieces during the day.*

> Exercise is youthing! Walk, cycle, jog on the spot while the kettle boils, bend from the waist while brushing your teeth... it all increases strength and flexibility.

YOUTHING PROTEINS

Many surprising foods contain protein – quinoa and amaranth, for example, are higher in protein per 100g than Brazil and macadamia nuts. For youthing purposes, try to get most of your protein from non-meat sources by including a variety of the foods listed here in your diet.

★ Grains (especially amaranth, buckwheat, oats, quinoa, rye, wheat)

★ Legumes (especially beans, lentils, tempeh, tofu)

★ Vegetable proteins from artichoke, asparagus, beetroot, broccoli, cauliflower, coriander, green beans, kale, okra, parsley, spinach, seaweed ...

★ Nuts and seeds (only a handful a day as they are high in fat/calories), nut milks, nut butters

★ Goat/sheep's milk and yoghurt and goat/sheep/buffalo's milk/cheese (about 2 tbsp per day as they are high in fat/calories)

★ Fish (four to five times a week – eat herring, mackerel, salmon, sardines, trout rather than larger fish such as tuna or swordfish, which bioaccumulate mercury and other heavy metals (see eating organic, pages 92–3)

★ Eggs (up to seven a week, unless you tend towards constipation)

★ If you want to eat meat, have one portion (75–100g) no more than once a week of grouse, pheasant, partridge, wild rabbit, organic free-range chicken/turkey, organic free-range lamb (limit to once a month) or organic lamb's liver (if you suffer from anaemia).

6 If you have a weight concern, plate yourself at mealtimes: use 22cm plates (measuring across the diameter of the base, not the raised sides), which are slightly smaller than typical 26cm dinner plates. For breakfast and soups, use bowls around 12cm wide/7cm high to 14cm wide/5cm high. For puddings, use shallower bowls – around 12cm wide to 4cm high. Eating is often about visual cues and habits: if the eye sees a full 22cm plateful, your body will feel happy not hungry after eating it, even though it contains less food than a 26cm plateful.

You can pile your plate with food, but once you've eaten it, know that that is it – there is nothing until the next mealtime. If you tend to overeat, this is a good way of measuring your total consumption and ensuring you eat mindfully.

* * *

GOOD WATER

★ Drink filtered tap water wherever possible, and use for boiling in kettles too. Carbon-activated jug filters are inexpensive and remove sediment, chlorine and rust but not healthy minerals such as potassium and calcium. Multi-stage filtration systems can also remove heavy metals such as lead, but are expensive and have to be fitted to your domestic water system by a professional. If you are worried about the quality of tap water in your home (it can be affected by old or rusting pipes), ask your local council to test it.

★ With bottled water, try to drink only from glass bottles (to avoid contaminants from plastic), sourced from an area near you (to avoid travel pollution). Don't drink from a plastic bottle that has been in the sun as chemicals and endocrine disruptors are prone to leaching from warm plastic.

★ Don't drink carbonated water if you are prone to gas or bloating.

★ Don't drink tonic water or commercial fruity/sugared waters: they don't cleanse the body and are high in calories.

★ Soda water contains sodium salts and carbon dioxide, so avoid.

* * *

7 Drink six to eight glasses or 1.5 litres of good quality water (see above) a day.

8 With a good breakfast, you should be able to get to lunch without a snack. But you might need something in the afternoon. Eat a piece of fruit or raw veg like carrot and peppers if that satisfies you (adding protein such as a handful of nuts or seeds makes it more filling), or take some portable snacks, such as Spicy Chickpeas (see page 136) and Youthing Nut Bars (see page 137) with you when you're on the move. Freshly made juice makes a good afternoon snack.

9 Become disciplined around food and try not to eat without thinking. Just because you're eating something healthy (fruit, dried fruit, nuts, seeds, health bars) doesn't mean you can eat as much of it as you like. Many healthy foods are high in calories. Listen to your body, and only ever eat to become two-thirds full, rather than overstuffed. But don't throw away any left over food: most of the **EYY** dishes can be saved for another meal. That way you won't feel guilty.

10 Treat yourself: but remember that 'treat' means once a week, not once a day. So have a few pieces of 80% chocolate, a coffee, a slice of cake once a week. People used to eat sugary treat foods only on special occasions such as birthdays, weddings, holidays. Aim to re-create that mindset.

DETOX YOUR KITCHEN

Before you start the **EYY Eating Plan**, go through your cupboards and remove the foods you won't be eating. Give them away or put them in a separate cupboard if family or housemates aren't following the **EYY Programme**.

Then look at how you store food: you need a cool, dark cupboard for oils, for example, as heat quickly turns oil rancid. Avoid keeping foods in cupboards with lights underneath – these generate a lot of heat, which spoils not just oils but nuts, grains and dried foods too.

As you'll be eating more fresh foods and vegetables, the fridge becomes the centre of the kitchen. Store delicate oils like flaxseed, sugar-free jam, tahini, nut butters and sprouted breads there, as well as some veg and fruit. Use a cold larder or cupboard to store the rest of your veg, fruit, beans, breads and condiments.

LOOK AFTER YOUR POTS AND PANS

It's important to choose pans and other cooking utensils that do not leach heavy metals or other contaminants into food. Here are some guidelines:

★ Only use heavy-based stainless-steel, cast-iron or copper pans with a stainless-steel finish inside. Avoid aluminium pans and any coated with Teflon or other non-stick finishes. Anodized aluminium pans can be used provided they are not scratched or damaged in any way.

★ Do not use pans with plastic handles, as they can emit toxic fumes when they are heated.

★ Use wooden spoons and spatulas to stir food rather than plastic or metal ones, which can leach contaminants or scratch the pan's surface.

★ If you cook or store food in enamelled or terracotta/glazed earthenware cookware, make sure you only use food safety approved brands as lead, cadmium and other heavy metals in the glazes may leach into food.

* * *

DRINKING YOUTHFULLY

Treat alcohol as a treat: that means an occasional glass, no more than once a week. Choose organic red wine rather than white, and if you want hard liquor, make it a small measure of good-quality vodka served with homemade juice (orange, lime, tomato).

* * *

The youthing larder

As well as being packed with a wide variety of fresh veg, herbs and fruit, the basic youthing larder may contain:

★ Beans and legumes: aduki beans, black beans, chickpeas, kidney beans, lentils, soya/edamame beans, split peas, sprouted beans (mung and alfafa).
★ Breads: homemade, rye and sprouted (from health food shops).
★ Dairy: only goat/sheep/buffalo's milk, cheese, yoghurt, butter or kefir.
★ Condiments: apple cider vinegar (organic, with mother – the cloudy bacterial culture that produces vinegar); flaxseed powder (cold-milled for omega-3s, sprinkle on salads or in juices); liquid aminos (add protein and salty flavour without fat or salt); miso (naturally fermented); nutritional yeast (adds flavour and B vitamins); seaweed (dulse, kombu, nori, wakame); soy sauce – no salt version only.
★ Dried fruits (unsulphured, unsweetened): apricots, dates, figs, goji berries, prunes, raisins.
★ Drinks: filtered water, herbal teas, homemade juices and smoothies.
★ Flour: barley, buckwheat, kamut, potato, rice, spelt.
★ Homemade Vegetable Stock (see page 142).
★ Miscellaneous: xanthum gum (rising agent); agar or vegetable flakes (for making jellies); Chinese mushrooms (shiitake, maitake, reishi for flavour and nutrients), dried or fresh; tempeh and tofu (for protein).
★ Nuts and seeds: almond, cashew, coconut, flaxseed, pistachio, pumpkin, sesame, sunflower, walnut. Nut and seed butters, tahini and nut milks.
★ Oils (untreated): almond, avocado, coconut, flaxseed, pumpkin, rapeseed, sesame oil.
★ Tinned foods: coconut milk (organic, without added sugar), tinned beans (organic, without added salt or sugar).
★ Whole grains: amaranth, black/brown rice, kamut, millet, oat groats, pearl barley, quinoa, rye, spelt, wheat.

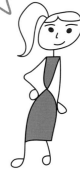

> If you want junk food, make it yourself – it's so much more youthing than anything you can buy ...

EATING ORGANIC

On the **EYY Eating Plan,** you're aiming to reduce your exposure to artificial food additives, pesticides and heavy metals, as these contain youth-robbing

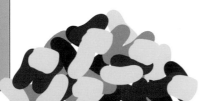

toxins that affect cellular functioning and may trigger inflammation. Plant foods grown organically also contain more minerals and antioxidants, according to a 2009 review by Denis Lairon of the University of Aix-Marseille. For those reasons, I'd like you to eat organic foods wherever you can.

However, organic foods can be expensive so if you are on a budget you need to make smart choices. Here are my organic tips:

1 Always try to buy organic apples, blueberries, celery, cherries, grapes, kale/collard greens, nectarines, peaches, peppers, root vegetables (carrots, parsnips, potatoes, etc.), spinach and strawberries, as these are contaminated with high levels of pesticides.

2 You don't need to buy organic asparagus, aubergine, avocado, cabbage, grapefruit, kiwi fruit, mango, melon, onions, peas, pineapple, sweetcorn or watermelon – these are the least contaminated by pesticides. If fruit and veg have a thick skin you remove before eating, such as bananas and oranges, it is generally fine to buy non-organic.

3 Don't buy organic fish – it is farmed and often full of fat, parasites and disease. (See also page 37 for more information about which fish to eat.)

4 If you are going to eat meat, try to buy organic, free-range, outdoor-bred varieties. Get it from a butcher or farm shop rather than a supermarket, as it is easier to trace its provenance.

FOODS TO AVOID

These foods will age you. Try not to have them in your kitchen or your life.

★ Processed and pre-packaged foods
★ White pasta, rice and flour products
★ Manufactured breakfast cereals
★ All fat-free or low-fat foods
★ Margarines, processed fats or anything containing trans-fats
★ Smoked or cured meats/fish
★ Any 'fresh' food with a shelf life of more than a month
★ Tinned foods with added salt and sweeteners
★ Sugar- or fat-loaded foods including confectionery and fried foods
★ Sweetened or artificially sweetened soft drinks and teas
★ All GM foods.

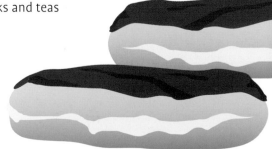

Foods to eat: the Youthing Food Chart

As well as the five best youthing foods, you ideally want to eat a wide variety of carbs, proteins and fats that help minimize the five ageing processes. Here is a detailed colour-coded chart outlining the healthy foods that help counter acidification, inflammation, oxidation, eliminative slowdown and hormonal imbalance. These are great youthing choices to incorporate into your diet.

You'll notice that meat and dairy are not listed. Although they contain protein they don't have any youthing benefits, so I have left them out. If a food you eat regularly is not on the chart (like yeast extract), the chances are that it has no youthing potential, so try to eat it less often and substitute something more youthing instead.

VEGETABLES	ANTI-INFLAMMATORY	ANTIOXIDANT	HORMONAL BALANCE	DIGESTIVE/ ELIMINATIVE	ALKALINE
Artichoke	✔	✔		✔	✔
Asian shoots/beansprouts/ bamboo shoots	✔	✔	✔		✔
Asparagus	✔	✔		✔	✔
Aubergine		✔	✔		✔
Barley grass	✔	✔	✔	✔	✔
Beetroot	✔	✔	✔	✔	✔
Bok choy/pak choi		✔			✔
Broad/fava beans	✔	✔	✔	✔	
Broccoli	✔	✔	✔	✔	✔
Brussels sprouts	✔	✔	✔	✔	✔
Cabbage red/white	✔	✔		✔	✔
Carrot	✔	✔	✔	✔	✔
Cauliflower	✔	✔		✔	✔
Celeriac	✔	✔		✔	✔
Celery	✔	✔		✔	✔
Chicory	✔	✔	✔	✔	✔
Chinese leaf (cabbage)	✔	✔	✔	✔	✔
Chinese mustard greens	✔	✔	✔	✔	✔
Courgette		✔			✔
Cucumber	✔	✔		✔	✔
Dandelion	✔	✔	✔	✔	✔
Daikon (white radish)			✔	✔	✔
Edible calendula	✔	✔		✔	✔
Endive		✔		✔	✔
Fennel	✔	✔	✔	✔	✔
Garlic	✔	✔	✔	✔	✔
Green beans	✔	✔	✔		✔

VEGETABLES	ANTI-INFLAMMATORY	ANTIOXIDANT	HORMONAL BALANCE	DIGESTIVE/ ELIMINATIVE	ALKALINE
Jerusalem artichoke	✔	✔		✔	✔
Kale/cavolo nero	✔	✔	✔	✔	✔
Leek	✔	✔		✔	✔
Lemongrass	✔	✔		✔	✔
Lettuce: iceberg, lamb's, romaine	✔	✔			✔
Lettuce: rocket, radicchio, chicory, curly endive	✔	✔		✔	✔
Mushroom: button, garden, portobello		✔		✔	
Mushroom: shiitake, maitake, umeboshi, reishi		✔	✔	✔	✔
Mustard greens	✔	✔		✔	✔
Okra	✔	✔	✔	✔	✔
Onion	✔	✔	✔	✔	✔
Parsnip		✔		✔	✔
Peas: garden peas, mangetout, petit pois, sugar peas	✔	✔	✔	✔	✔
Pepper: bell/sweet		✔	✔		✔
Potato	✔	✔		✔	✔
Pumpkin	✔	✔		✔	✔
Radish	✔	✔	✔	✔	✔
Seaweed: dulse, kombo, nori, samphire, wakame	✔	✔	✔	✔	✔
Sorrel	✔	✔		✔	✔
Spinach	✔	✔		✔	✔
Spring onions/scallions	✔	✔	✔	✔	✔
Sprouts	✔	✔	✔	✔	✔
Squash, butternut	✔	✔		✔	✔
Swede (rutabaga)	✔	✔		✔	✔
Sweet potato/yam	✔	✔	✔	✔	✔
Sweetcorn		✔		✔	✔
Swiss chard	✔	✔		✔	✔
Turnip	✔	✔		✔	✔
Water chestnut	✔	✔		✔	✔
Watercress	✔	✔		✔	✔
Wheatgrass	✔	✔		✔	✔
FRUIT					
Apple		✔	✔	✔	✔
Apricot		✔	✔	✔	✔
Avocado	✔	✔	✔	✔	✔
Banana	✔	✔	✔	✔	✔
Blackberry/dewberry	✔	✔	✔	✔	✔
Blackcurrant/red/pink/ white currant	✔	✔	✔	✔	
Blueberry/bilberry	✔	✔	✔	✔	✔
Cherry	✔	✔	✔	✔	✔
Coconut (fresh)	✔	✔		✔	✔
Cranberry	✔	✔	✔	✔	

FRUIT CONT.	ANTI-INFLAMMATORY	ANTIOXIDANT	HORMONAL BALANCE	DIGESTIVE/ ELIMINATIVE	ALKALINE
Date	✔	✔	✔	✔	✔
Fig (fresh)		✔	✔	✔	✔
Grapefruit	✔	✔	✔	✔	✔
Grape: black, red, white	✔	✔		✔	✔
Goji berry	✔	✔	✔	✔	✔
Gooseberry: green, red	✔	✔	✔	✔	
Kiwi fruit	✔	✔		✔	✔
Lemon	✔	✔		✔	✔
Lime	✔	✔		✔	✔
Lychee	✔	✔	✔	✔	✔
Mandarin/satsuma/ tangerine	✔	✔		✔	✔
Mango		✔		✔	✔
Melon/watermelon	✔	✔	✔	✔	✔
Mulberry	✔	✔		✔	✔
Olive	✔	✔	✔	✔	✔
Orange	✔	✔		✔	✔
Papaya	✔	✔	✔	✔	✔
Passion fruit	✔	✔		✔	✔
Peach/nectarine	✔	✔		✔	✔
Pear	✔	✔		✔	✔
Pineapple	✔	✔		✔	✔
Plum/damson/greengage	✔	✔		✔	✔
Pomegranate	✔	✔	✔	✔	✔
Prune		✔	✔	✔	✔
Raisins		✔		✔	✔
Raspberry/cloudberry	✔	✔	✔	✔	✔
Rhubarb		✔	✔	✔	✔
Strawberry	✔	✔	✔	✔	✔
Tomato		✔	✔	✔	✔
GRAINS					
Amaranth	✔	✔		✔	✔
Barley: pearl	✔	✔	✔	✔	✔
Buckwheat	✔	✔	✔		✔
Chickpea, lentil or soya flour		✔	✔	✔	✔
Corn		✔	✔		
Hemp	✔	✔	✔	✔	
Kamut/durum wheat		✔	✔		
Millet	✔	✔	✔	✔	✔
Oats	✔	✔	✔	✔	
Quinoa	✔	✔	✔		✔
Rice: black, red	✔	✔	✔	✔	✔
Rice: brown	✔	✔	✔	✔	
Rye	✔	✔	✔	✔	✔
Sorghum	✔	✔			
Soy lecithin	✔	✔	✔	✔	✔
Spelt	✔	✔			
Sprouted grains	✔		✔	✔	
Wheat (whole)	✔	✔	✔		

LEGUMES	ANTI-INFLAMMATORY	ANTIOXIDANT	HORMONAL BALANCE	DIGESTIVE/ ELIMINATIVE	ALKALINE
Aduki beans/azuki	✔	✔	✔	✔	✔
Alfalfa sprouts	✔	✔	✔	✔	✔
Black beans	✔	✔	✔	✔	✔
Borlotti beans	✔	✔	✔	✔	✔
Broad/fava beans	✔	✔	✔	✔	
Butter beans	✔	✔	✔	✔	✔
Cannellini beans	✔	✔	✔	✔	✔
Chickpeas		✔	✔	✔	
Haricot verts	✔	✔		✔	
Kidney beans	✔	✔	✔	✔	✔
Lentils: green, brown, red, Puy, split	✔	✔	✔	✔	
Miso	✔	✔	✔	✔	✔
Mung beans	✔	✔	✔	✔	✔
Peas: green, yellow, split	✔	✔	✔	✔	
Pinto beans	✔	✔	✔	✔	✔
Soya/edamame beans	✔	✔	✔	✔	✔
Tempeh/tofu			✔		✔
NUTS & SEEDS					
Almond	✔	✔	✔	✔	✔
Anise seeds	✔	✔	✔	✔	✔
Brazil	✔	✔	✔	✔	
Cashew	✔	✔	✔		
Chestnut	✔	✔	✔		✔
Coconut	✔	✔	✔	✔	✔
Flaxseeds/linseeds	✔	✔	✔	✔	✔
Hazelnut	✔	✔	✔		✔
Macadamia	✔	✔	✔	✔	
Nut butters	✔	✔	✔	✔	
Peanut, unsalted		✔	✔		
Pecan	✔	✔	✔		
Pine nut	✔	✔	✔		
Pistachio		✔	✔	✔	
Pumpkin seeds	✔	✔	✔	✔	✔
Sesame seeds	✔	✔	✔	✔	✔
Sprouted seeds	✔	✔		✔	✔
Sunflower seeds	✔	✔	✔	✔	✔
Tahini	✔	✔	✔	✔	✔
Walnut	✔	✔	✔		
Water chestnut	✔	✔	✔	✔	✔
HERBS & SPICES					
Basil	✔	✔	✔	✔	✔
Black pepper	✔	✔		✔	✔
Cardamom	✔		✔	✔	✔
Cayenne	✔	✔		✔	✔
Chilli	✔	✔		✔	✔
Chive	✔			✔	✔

HERBS & SPICES CONT.	ANTI-INFLAMMATORY	ANTIOXIDANT	HORMONAL BALANCE	DIGESTIVE/ELIMINATIVE	ALKALINE
Cinnamon	✔	✔	✔	✔	✔
Cloves	✔	✔		✔	✔
Coriander	✔	✔	✔	✔	✔
Cumin	✔	✔		✔	✔
Curry leaf	✔	✔		✔	✔
Dill	✔	✔	✔	✔	✔
Ginger	✔	✔		✔	✔
Horseradish	✔	✔		✔	✔
Mint	✔	✔		✔	✔
Mustard (yellow) seed	✔	✔		✔	✔
Nutmeg	✔	✔	✔	✔	✔
Oregano/marjoram	✔	✔	✔	✔	✔
Parsley	✔	✔	✔	✔	✔
Rosemary	✔	✔	✔	✔	✔
Saffron	✔	✔		✔	✔
Sage	✔	✔	✔	✔	✔
Tamarind	✔	✔	✔	✔	✔
Tarragon	✔			✔	✔
Thyme	✔	✔			✔
Turmeric	✔	✔	✔	✔	✔
Vanilla pod	✔			✔	✔
Wasabi	✔	✔		✔	✔
FISH					
Brill	✔	✔			
Cod	✔	✔			
Crab		✔	✔		
Dover sole	✔	✔			
Haddock	✔	✔			
Halibut	✔	✔			
Herring	✔	✔			
John Dory	✔	✔			
Lemon sole	✔	✔			
Lobster		✔	✔		
Mahimahi	✔	✔			
Monkfish	✔	✔			
Mullet, red	✔	✔			
Oysters		✔	✔		
Plaice	✔	✔			
Sardines/pilchards	✔	✔			
Salmon	✔	✔			
Scallops		✔			
Snapper, red	✔	✔			
Swordfish	✔	✔			
Trout	✔	✔			
Tuna	✔	✔			
Whitebait	✔	✔			
EGGS					
Chicken, duck, quail			✔		

SWEETENERS	ANTI-INFLAMMATORY	ANTIOXIDANT	HORMONAL BALANCE	DIGESTIVE/ELIMINATIVE	ALKALINE
Blackstrap molasses		✔	✔	✔	
Fresh fruit juice, reduced		✔		✔	
Honey, unrefined	✔	✔	✔	✔	
Sweet apricot paste	✔	✔	✔	✔	✔

MISCELLANEOUS	ANTI-INFLAMMATORY	ANTIOXIDANT	HORMONAL BALANCE	DIGESTIVE/ELIMINATIVE	ALKALINE
Apple cider vinegar (with mother)	✔	✔		✔	✔
Chocolate, 80%+		✔	✔		
Liquid aminos			✔		
Probiotic culture	✔			✔	
Salt, Himalayan/mineral	✔	✔	✔		
Sugar-free jam		✔			
Veg stock, homemade, no salt	✔	✔		✔	✔

DRINKS	ANTI-INFLAMMATORY	ANTIOXIDANT	HORMONAL BALANCE	DIGESTIVE/ELIMINATIVE	ALKALINE
Apple juice, unsweetened	✔	✔		✔	
Coconut juice, from fresh	✔	✔	✔	✔	✔
Coconut milk	✔	✔	✔		✔
Coffee, dandelion	✔	✔	✔	✔	
Cranberry juice, unsweetened	✔	✔			
Fruit tea		✔		✔	
Grape juice	✔	✔		✔	
Orange juice (freshly squeezed)	✔	✔		✔	✔
Red wine, organic		✔			
Tea: black, green, herbal	✔	✔			
Tomato juice		✔			
Soya milk		✔	✔	✔	✔
Vegetable juice, fresh	✔	✔	✔	✔	✔

COLD-PRESSED OILS	ANTI-INFLAMMATORY	ANTIOXIDANT	HORMONAL BALANCE	DIGESTIVE/ELIMINATIVE	ALKALINE
Almond oil	✔	✔		✔	✔
Avocado oil	✔	✔	✔		✔
Borage oil	✔	✔			✔
Coconut oil	✔	✔		✔	✔
Evening primrose oil	✔	✔	✔	✔	✔
Grapeseed oil	✔	✔			✔
Hemp oil	✔	✔	✔		
Flaxseed/linseed oil	✔	✔	✔	✔	✔
Hazelnut oil		✔			✔
Olive oil	✔	✔	✔	✔	✔
Peanut oil	✔	✔			
Pumpkin oil	✔	✔	✔		✔
Rapeseed oil	✔	✔			✔
Rice bran oil	✔	✔			
Sesame oil	✔	✔	✔		✔
Sunflower oil	✔				✔
Walnut oil	✔		✔		

Basic cooking tips

It helps if you can neatly organize your kitchen so things are at your fingertips instead of having to wade through cupboards to find them, and also if you have a few important kitchen basics like the pastes, dried tomatoes, vegetable stock and almond milk to hand (see pages 142–7 for recipes).

STEAM FRYING

Some ways of cooking foods are more youthing than others – steam frying is low in fat but retains all the flavour. It's easy to do:

Store your food in glass containers. Plastic contains molecules that can act as endocrine disruptors, mimicking the effects of oestrogen and other hormones. Don't let cling-film touch your food, and don't use it to cover food that is still hot.

1 Put a heavy-based frying pan or saucepan on a medium heat for a few minutes until hot but not smoking.

2 Put ½ tsp of oil (preferably coconut oil) into the pan, to coat it and prevent sticking.

3 Add 4–6 tbsp of water (more if you need it). Wait until the water is bubbling and steaming, then add onions, garlic or whatever food you are steam frying. Cook as normal.

SPROUTING BEANS AND SEEDS

It takes a few days to sprout your own beans and seeds but the process is very easy with a commercial sprouting jar or large glass jar. Use seeds or small beans – dried organic aduki or mung beans are perfect – as larger beans taste bitter when sprouted. Rinse well, place in the jar covered with water, cover with muslin (fix it with a rubber band) and soak for 12–24 hours. Pour out the water, discard any hard beans/seeds, rinse again, then spread them out in the muslin-covered jar and leave to sprout at room temperature out of direct sunlight. Rinse twice a day for the next 2–4 days (depending on the size you like to eat them). Harvest, rinse and pat dry, and they'll keep in the fridge for up to a week.

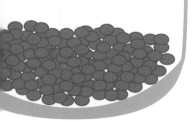

COOKING DRIED BEANS

It's vital to cook beans properly as they can be toxic if you don't. The best way is to soak them overnight – they'll take much less time to cook. Beans yield around two to three times their original volume. You don't need to soak lentils.

Overnight soak method: put the beans in a bowl, cover with water and leave to soak overnight or for at least 8 hours in the fridge to discourage fermentation. The next day, discard any beans which are floating, rinse the rest and put in a pan with around three to four times as much water. Do not add salt or other flavourings. Bring to the boil and boil for 10 minutes. Skim off any foam. Then turn down the heat to a simmer and cook uncovered for the following times: black-eyed beans, cannellini beans – about 45 minutes; aduki beans – around 50 minutes; butter, kidney beans – around 1 hour; black, pinto beans – 1½ hours; chickpeas – around 2 hours; soya beans – around 3 hours. The beans should be firm, but cooked through. Drain. Use the bean cooking water as a stock as it contains many nutrients.

Quick soak method: add ¼ tsp of bicarbonate of soda for each cup of beans, cover with water and boil for 2 minutes. Set aside to soak for an hour. Then rinse off the water, add around three to four times as much water as beans, bring back to the boil and then simmer until ready (see times above). Quick soak beans tend to be slightly mushier than those soaked overnight.

SEEDS, NUTS AND DRIED FRUITS

Blanch these in boiling water for a minute before eating – it helps kill surface bacteria. For best youthing results, soak nuts overnight to help activate enzymes. Nuts and seeds have a high oil content, and can quickly go rancid. Pick them over before using, discarding any that are discoloured, limp or musty. Rather than buying crushed or sliced nuts, prepare your own from whole nuts, they

* * *

EASY PEELING

Almonds: put them in boiling water for 30 minutes and the skins will slide off when you rub them.

Squash can be tough to peel. If you heat the whole squash in the oven for a few minutes, the skin comes off more easily.

Tomatoes: a quick, easy way to peel tomatoes is to place them whole in a heatproof bowl, then cover with boiling water. Leave for a minute or two, and the skins will split. You can then slide them off with your fingers (plunge the tomatoes into cold water if they are too hot to touch).

* * *

After 6 days on the **EYY Eating Plan**, your taste buds will change – you'll find very sweet or salty foods an assault on the senses ...

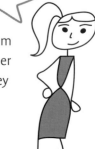

will be fresher. Store seeds, nuts and dried fruits in a cool, dry place in airtight containers, and eat within 3 months of purchase.

COOKING OAT GROATS

Delicious, nutty and nutritious, eat oat groats instead of rolled oats for breakfast. For best results, soak in freshly boiled water for 1 hour (or overnight). Drain the water then put the oats in a pan with fresh water and simmer for about 20 minutes. You can add cinnamon for a warming, satisfying breakfast which is more blood-sugar stabilizing than milled oats. If time is short in the morning, you can also cook them in the evening and reheat the next morning.

JUICERS
TO MAKE VEGETABLE JUICES, YOU WILL NEED A JUICER. IT MAKES THE JOB SIMPLE AND QUICK – A JOY NOT A CHORE. LOOK FOR A JUICER WITH A WIDE MOUTH (SO YOU DON'T HAVE TO CHOP FRUIT AND VEG UP SMALL) THAT IS EASY TO CLEAN. SOME PEOPLE ARGUE ABOUT THE BENEFITS OF CENTRIFUGAL VERSUS COLD-PRESS JUICERS – THE LATTER IS MORE YOUTHING AS ENZYMES ARE NOT DESTROYED BY HEAT, BUT THEY ARE MUCH MORE EXPENSIVE.

JUICING

Drinking raw juice every morning is the most fabulous youthing start to the day. There is no quicker way to get a powerhouse of live enzymes, minerals, vitamins and other phytonutrients into your body. Juicing helps raise energy levels and boost immunity, making you look and feel brighter, more youthful, more vibrant. It's also delicious and possibly borderline addictive – especially if you whack in the ginger, lemon, mint and other fresh herbs.

Drinking raw, freshly made juice helps accelerate all five youthing aims. Veg and fruit are naturally alkalizing, antioxidant, anti-inflammatory and detoxifying. Juice is intensely packed with enzymes that promote the regeneration of cells, tissues and organs, and regulate metabolism, affecting weight loss. Juices are considered to provide more bioavailable minerals than the original raw veg or fruit – the act of juicing releases minerals such as calcium and potassium from hard-to-digest fibre so we can absorb them more easily. Juicing is also a great way to get three of the best youthing foods – beetroot, turmeric and lemon – into your diet and, if you're brave, you can pop in a garlic clove too.

* * *

HOW TO START JUICING

★ The produce you use should be fresh and ideally organic. If not, you can use a veggie wash to remove surface pesticides and other contaminants. Wash all produce before juicing to remove surface bacteria. Peel where necessary (for example, beetroot and ginger). You don't need to core apples or peel lemons.

★ Do a bulk buy of juicing produce every 5 days, so you always have something reasonably fresh to hand. Don't juice heavily bruised or damaged produce, but do juice the outer leaves – these are often highest in nutrients.

★ The most cleansing veg/herbs are basil, beetroot, carrot, celery, cucumber, ginger, parsley, radish, spinach, watercress. The most cleansing fruit are apple, grapes, lemon, pear and watermelon.

★ You can add other nutrients to your juice – for example, powdered flaxseeds, soya, rice or pea protein powder or amino acid powder (from health food shops).

★ Make small quantities of juice and drink it as soon as you have made it – raw juices lose their potency quickly.

★ Keep veg in the fridge so your juice comes out tasting cool and refreshing. In summer, you can also add a couple of ice cubes (made with filtered water) to the liquidizer or juicer.

★ Apples, pears and lemons mix well with veg juices, but other fruits are best kept separate.

★ Start small – try apple and carrot first, add ginger and lemon, then kale, spinach, beetroot and whatever else takes your fancy.

★ Work up towards drinking a big glass (around 250–300ml) of veg juice at least once a day. Juices make good afternoon snacks too.

★ Remember to chew your juice, drink slowly and swirl round the mouth for maximum benefit.

* * *

Cleansing and rejuvenating juices

Each of these juices makes 1 glass, unless stated otherwise. Making them couldn't be easier: prepare all the ingredients, push through a juicer and drink at once. For more juicing tips, see pages 102–3.

 ## WATERCRESS, BEETROOT & CARROT ZINGER

This is a super-youthing, vitamin-rich juice. Stir the turmeric into the juiced vegetables and apple.

- ★ 50g watercress, trimmed
- ★ 2 raw baby beetroot, peeled and cut into wedges
- ★ 2 large carrots, peeled
- ★ 1 celery stick, trimmed and roughly chopped
- ★ 1 apple
- ★ ¼ tsp turmeric

 ## DETOX ROOT & BEETROOT BURST

Packed with root veg for a classic cleansing hit. Stir the turmeric into the juiced vegetables, adding more lemon if you want a sharper taste.

- ★ 1 small turnip, peeled
- ★ 1 large or 2 small raw beetroot, peeled
- ★ 1 parsnip, peeled
- ★ 2 large carrots, peeled
- ★ 5 radishes
- ★ 1 organic lemon
- ★ ¼ tsp turmeric

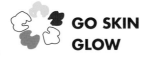 ## GO SKIN GLOW

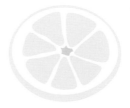

Full of betacarotene to help skin glow.

- ★ 1 sweet potato, peeled and roughly chopped
- ★ 3 carrots, peeled
- ★ 1 white turnip, peeled and roughly chopped
- ★ 1 lemon
- ★ Thumbnail of fresh root ginger, peeled

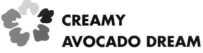 ## CREAMY AVOCADO DREAM

This deliciously creamy juice – thanks to the avocado – ticks all five of my youthing boxes. Juice the celery, lemon, parsley and kale first, then pour into a liquidizer and blend with the avocado and oregano.

- ★ 1 celery stick, trimmed
- ★ 1 lemon
- ★ Handful parsley
- ★ 6 kale leaves or 2 small handfuls curly kale
- ★ ½ avocado, peeled and stoned
- ★ Sprig of oregano, chopped

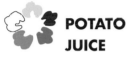 ## POTATO JUICE

Drinking potato juice in the morning can help constipation – but don't drink the sediment or use green or sprouting potatoes.

- ★ 1 potato, peeled
- ★ 1 carrot, peeled
- ★ ½ apple

 ## APPLE & CARROT DETOX SPEEDER

A sweet and tangy juice for cleansing the digestive system.

- ★ ¼ white cabbage, roughly chopped
- ★ 3–4 carrots, peeled
- ★ 1 small apple
- ★ 5cm fresh root ginger, peeled

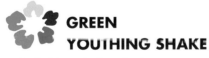 ## GREEN YOUTHING SHAKE

Full of chlorophyll and other green goodies, this is one of my top all-round youthers. Add lemon if you want to sharpen the taste.

- ★ Handful parsley
- ★ Handful kale
- ★ Handful spinach
- ★ ½ green pepper
- ★ 1 celery stick, trimmed
- ★ ½ lemon (optional)

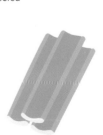

SUPER-CHARGED SPRING CLEANER

Good for detox and digestion, and packed with vitamins and minerals to give a youthing boost.

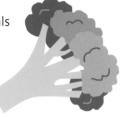

- ★ 2 carrots, peeled
- ★ 1 beetroot, peeled
- ★ 5cm fresh root ginger, peeled
- ★ 1 apple
- ★ 3 florets broccoli
- ★ ½ lemon

 ## PEPPY VIRGIN MARY

Highly antioxidant, this also helps stimulate the digestive system.

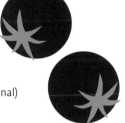

- ★ 4 tomatoes
- ★ ½ lemon
- ★ 1 celery stick, trimmed
- ★ 3 radishes, trimmed
- ★ 1 slice horseradish root (optional)

1 Put the tomatoes, lemon, celery and radishes through a juicer.
2 Carefully peel the horseradish (wash your hands immediately after – it can make your eyes and nose run), then juice that too. Drink at once.

 ## PEAR & FIG WINTER SMOOTHIE

A sweet, creamy, warming winter drink.

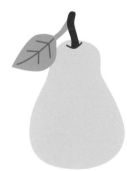

MAKES 2 GLASSES

- ★ 2 pears, peeled, cored and roughly chopped
- ★ 2 fresh figs, topped, tailed and roughly chopped
- ★ 480ml Almond Milk (see page 147)

1 Blend or process all the ingredients until smooth. Pour into glasses and drink.

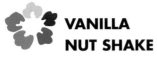 ## VANILLA NUT SHAKE

A rich, creamy smoothie full of nutty flavour that will keep for 3–4 days in the fridge.

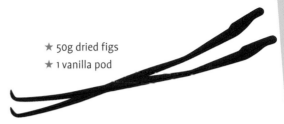

MAKES 4 GLASSES

★ 30g almonds
★ 20g Brazil nuts
★ 30g macadamia nuts
★ 20g sesame seeds
★ 50g dried figs
★ 1 vanilla pod

1 Soak the nuts and seeds in cold water for at least 1 hour. Drain them and put in a liquidizer with 1 litre water and whiz until smooth.
2 Blanch the figs for a minute in boiling water. Drain.
3 Split the vanilla pod down its length, scrape out the seeds and discard the pod.
4 Add the figs and vanilla seeds to the blended nuts and seeds and whiz until smooth. This gives a thick, wholesome smoothie, but you can strain it if you wish.
5 Store the smoothie in the fridge.

 ## GOLDEN CHAI

A traditional Indian recipe for bringing down inflammation – I've used dates as a sweetener instead of honey.

MAKES 2 GLASSES

★ ½ tsp Youthing Turmeric Paste (see page 146)
★ 2 Medjool dates, chopped into quarters
★ 1 tsp almond oil
★ 200ml Almond Milk (see page 117)

1 Put the turmeric paste, dates and almond oil in a pan and stir well.
2 Over a low to medium heat, slowly stir the Almond Milk into the paste mixture. Heat until just below boiling point.
3 Remove the dates (you can eat them separately) with a slotted spoon, then aerate the milk until it is frothy to heighten its flavour – you can blend it, whisk it or pour it between 2 containers held at arm's length. Drink while still warm.

Breakfast

I love breakfast, it's the most creative meal of the day. Yet many people can't face eating first thing in the morning – the trouble is that by 11am they find themselves two lattes and a muffin down. It's much better to eat a decent breakfast of complex carbs, protein and fruit that will sustain you without snacking until lunch. That might typically be: a small bowl of porridge or homemade cereal with nut milk, and two slices of toast with fruit or homemade no-sugar jam. Or an egg, homemade Baked Beans (see below) or mushrooms on toast, with a piece of fruit. Or fruity muesli and goat's yoghurt, with a slice of nutty toast. Occasionally, if you have a craving for something sweet, eat a piece of cake, scone or pud (from an **EYY** recipe), or a serving of Creamy Coconut & Pineapple Black Rice Pud (see page 131), with fruit and a slice of toast and cereal. However, if eating sweet things makes you sluggish, omit until your body can handle it. There are lots of other breakfast ideas in the detox chapter (see pages 82–4).

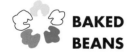 **BAKED BEANS**

Eat on toast with mushrooms and poached egg for breakfast, or as a side dish later in the day with a baked potato. They will keep in the fridge for about 4 days.

MAKES 1 GENEROUS PORTION

- ★ 1 tomato, finely chopped
- ★ 4 oven-dried tomatoes with oil, finely chopped
- ★ ½ tin cannellini beans (or more if wanted)
- ★ 1 pinch mineral salt
- ★ ½ tsp nutritional yeast
- ★ Pepper or harissa paste (optional)

1 Put the fresh and dried tomatoes in a dry frying pan and slowly heat until the skin on the tomato has fallen off, the tomato has fallen apart and the dried tomato has become part of the paste. Put into a liquidizer with 240ml water and blend until fine.

2 Place the mixture in a saucepan with the cannellini beans, salt and nutritional yeast and simmer for 15 minutes until almost all the water has reduced, but there is a nice creamy sauce.

3 Season with pepper, if you want, or add a little harissa paste to make it spicy.

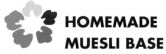

HOMEMADE MUESLI BASE

Add fresh fruit, yoghurt and/or Almond Milk (see page 147) to give a substantial, filling breakfast that ticks all five youthing boxes. This muesli also makes a delicious fruit crumble topping and filling for baked apples (see page 110). It will last for 1 week in an airtight container.

MAKES 2 PORTIONS

- ★ 15g sunflower seeds
- ★ 15g pumpkin seeds
- ★ 25g walnuts
- ★ 25g almonds
- ★ 10g dried unsulphured apricots
- ★ 75g porridge oats

1 Blanch the seeds, nuts and apricots in boiling water for 2 minutes. Drain and pat dry on a clean tea towel. Roughly chop the almonds, walnuts and apricots.
2 Mix all the ingredients together.

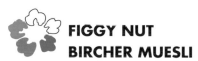

FIGGY NUT BIRCHER MUESLI

Make this the night before and leave in the fridge to bring out the spicy undertones. You can add fresh fruit, such as apple, banana or berries, before serving. It will keep for 2 days.

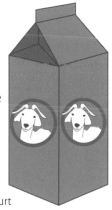

MAKES 2 BOWLS

- ★ 4 dried figs
- ★ 150g rolled oats
- ★ 160ml goat's milk
- ★ 160ml orange juice, freshly squeezed
- ★ 200g goat/sheep's yoghurt
- ★ ½ tsp ground cinnamon
- ★ 70g chopped walnuts

1 Plunge the figs into boiling water for 30 seconds, then rinse under cold running water. Chop roughly.
2 Combine the figs with the oats, milk, juice, yoghurt, cinnamon and half the nuts in a large bowl. Cover and refrigerate overnight.
3 Next morning, serve the muesli with the remaining nuts sprinkled over and fresh fruit, if using.

BUCKWHEAT PANCAKES WITH PEAR, APPLE & BLUEBERRY COMPOTE

A tasty, antioxidant-rich breakfast/brunch.

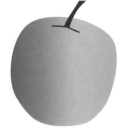

MAKES 5 SMALL PANCAKES

FOR THE PANCAKES
- ★ 50g buckwheat flour, sifted
- ★ ¼ tsp ground cinnamon, sifted
- ★ 1 egg
- ★ 150ml Almond Milk (see page 147)
- ★ ¼ tsp coconut oil, for frying

FOR THE COMPOTE
- ★ 1 apple, peeled, cored and thinly sliced
- ★ 1 pear, peeled, cored and thinly sliced
- ★ 100g blueberries (or blackberries when in season)

1 To make the pancakes, put the flour and cinnamon into a bowl. Make a well in the centre and add the egg and some of the milk. Whisk slowly, drawing in the flour. Whisk in the rest of the milk until you have a thin pancake batter with no lumps.
2 Heat a drop of oil in a small frying pan over a medium heat. Add a ladleful of batter and leave to cook until bubbles break on the surface, then turn. Cook for 1–2 minutes until golden. Put on a plate and cover to keep warm. Repeat until all the batter is used.
3 To make the compote, put the apple and pear slices in a small pan with 100ml water. Gently stew over a low heat until the fruit softens but holds its shape. Just before you're ready to serve, add the blueberries and stew for a further 2 minutes.
4 Place a pancake on a plate, spoon over some compote, roll and serve.

MUESLI BAKED APPLES

Serve on its own or with Vanilla Soya Custard (see page 133) as a dessert. The Muesli Base recipe is on page 109.

SERVES 4

- ★ 50g Homemade Muesli Base
- ★ 2 Medjool dates, finely chopped
- ★ ⅓ tbsp coconut oil
- ★ 2 tbsp blueberries
- ★ 4 large Granny Smith or Pink Lady apples, cored

1 Preheat the oven to 180°C/gas mark 4. Mix the muesli, dates, oil and blueberries in a bowl and stir to form a loose paste. Stuff the apples with the muesli mix until full.
2 Place on a baking tray and cook, uncovered, for 30–40 minutes until soft.

Soups and salads

Soups are great if you are trying to lose weight. They make you feel fuller for up to 1½ hours longer than solid food by slowing down the release of ghrelin, the hormone in the stomach walls that triggers the hunger pangs that make you want to eat more. Even better, cooking soups from fresh makes them hugely nutritious and youthing: pack in as many age-busting foods as you like. Try adding half an avocado, some goat's cheese or 1 tsp of coconut oil for extra creaminess. It's worth knowing that packaged (even healthy sounding varieties), tinned and soups in restaurants are often loaded with salt and other additives, so you may want to avoid them.

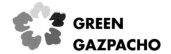 **GREEN GAZPACHO**

Fresh, light and cleansing, this energizing summer soup has a slight kick of chilli.

SERVES 4

- ★ 2 cucumbers, peeled and sliced
- ★ 1 romaine lettuce, roughly chopped
- ★ 4 celery sticks, trimmed and chopped
- ★ 4 spring onions, trimmed and chopped
- ★ 1 garlic clove, peeled and crushed
- ★ 1 heaped tsp chopped medium-hot green chilli
- ★ 1 avocado, peeled and stoned
- ★ 1 tsp lemon juice
- ★ 100g baby spinach
- ★ 15g mint leaves
- ★ 15g parsley, plus extra to garnish
- ★ A little avocado oil, to garnish

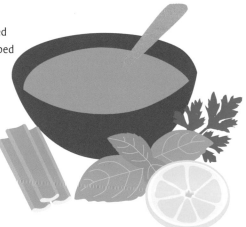

1 Put the cucumbers, lettuce, celery, spring onions, garlic, chilli pepper, avocado and lemon juice in a liquidizer and whiz until smooth. Add the spinach, mint and the 15g parsley for a brief whiz at the end.
2 Serve in bowls with a swirl of avocado oil and a little finely chopped parsley on top. Eat straightaway although it will keep in the fridge for 24 hours.

FENNEL SOUP

Fennel is rich in Vitamin C, potassium and other minerals. The soup is delicious served with Pumpkin Seed & Tomato Bread or Walnut Bread (see pages 138 and 139).

SERVES 4

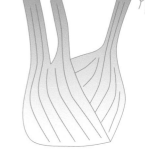

- ★ ½ tsp coconut oil
- ★ 1 onion, peeled and roughly chopped
- ★ 2 garlic cloves, peeled and roughly chopped
- ★ 2 fennel bulbs, trimmed and cut into 2cm cubes
- ★ 1 tsp fennel seeds
- ★ 1 litre homemade Vegetable Stock (see page 142)

1 Heat the oil in a saucepan over a gentle heat. Add the onion and garlic with 4–6 tbsp water and steam fry (see page 100) until soft.

2 Stir in the fennel and seeds and leave to steam fry for 5–10 minutes, stirring from time to time. If necessary, add a little more water to prevent sticking.

3 Add the stock and leave to simmer for a further 20 minutes. Allow to cool slightly then blend in a liquidizer until smooth.

 ## CREAMY BEETROOT DETOX SOUP

I love the intense, earthy flavours of this cleansing soup. Serve with any of the breads on pages 138–9 or crispbreads. It will keep for 4 days in the fridge, or freeze for up to 3 months.

SERVES 4

- ★ ½ tsp coconut oil
- ★ 1 small onion, peeled and roughly chopped
- ★ 4 celery sticks, trimmed and chopped
- ★ 1 apple, peeled, cored and chopped
- ★ 1 litre homemade Vegetable Stock (see page 142)
- ★ 4 raw beetroot, peeled and chopped

1 Heat the oil in a saucepan over a gentle heat. Add the onion with 4–6 tbsp water and steam fry (see page 100) until soft. Then add the celery, beetroot and apple and continue to steam fry for 5–10 minutes.

2 Add the stock, bring to the boil and simmer for 10 minutes or until the vegetables are cooked. If needed, add extra stock or water. Blend in a liquidizer until smooth.

ALKALIZING CANNELLINI BEAN SOUP

A meal in itself – packed with delicious, nutrient-rich veg. The soup is best eaten at once, but it will keep in the fridge for 2–3 days.

SERVES 6

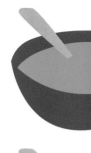

- ★ 115g pearl barley
- ★ Seaweed: choose from kombu (2 strips); wakame (1 tbsp); dulse (1 tbsp); or samphire (1 tbsp)
- ★ ½ tsp coconut oil
- ★ 1 onion, peeled and chopped
- ★ 2 garlic cloves, peeled and chopped
- ★ 1 potato, peeled and finely cubed
- ★ 1 sweet potato, peeled and finely cubed
- ★ 1 courgette, finely cubed

- ★ 1 carrot, peeled and finely cubed
- ★ 1 raw beetroot, peeled and finely cubed
- ★ 2 large tomatoes, peeled (see page 101) and roughly chopped
- ★ 1 litre homemade Vegetable Stock (see page 147)
- ★ 2 bay leaves
- ★ ½ tsp thyme
- ★ 400g tin cannellini beans
- ★ 1 tsp chopped parsley
- ★ 1 tsp chopped coriander

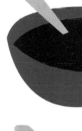

1 Put the pearl barley into a small saucepan and cover with cold water. Bring to the boil, then reduce the heat and simmer for about 20 minutes, stirring occasionally, until soft but with a bite. Add more water during cooking if needed. Drain and rinse under cold running water and set aside.

2 Soak the seaweed in water for 10–15 minutes (or follow the instructions on the packet).

3 Heat the oil in a saucepan over a gentle heat. Add the onion and garlic with 4–6 tbsp water and steam fry (see page 100) for about 5 minutes until soft.

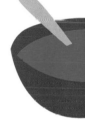

4 Add the potato, sweet potato, courgette, carrot, beetroot and tomatoes to the onion and stir to combine. Steam fry for a further 5–10 minutes, stirring occasionally.

5 Add the stock with the seaweed, bay leaves and thyme, cover and leave to simmer for about 20 minutes.

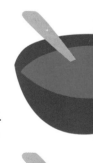

6 Add the pearl barley and drained, rinsed beans and continue to cook on a low heat for another 5 minutes. Remove the bay leaves and seaweed (unless using samphire).

7 Sprinkle the parsley and coriander on top before serving.

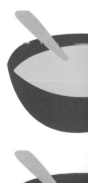

YOUTHING BUTTERNUT SQUASH & GINGER SOUP

Sweet and creamy with a fresh ginger tang, this is a great dinner party starter served with Walnut Bread (see page 139). It will keep in the fridge for 3 days.

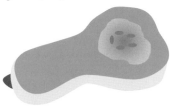

SERVES 4

★ ½ tsp coconut oil
★ 1 small onion, peeled and chopped
★ 1 garlic clove, peeled and crushed
★ 2cm fresh root ginger, peeled and finely chopped
★ ¾ small butternut squash, peeled, de-seeded and chopped into 1cm cubes
★ 1 litre homemade Vegetable Stock (see page 142)

1 Heat the oil in a saucepan over a gentle heat. Add the onion, garlic and ginger with 4–6 tbsp water and steam fry (see page 100) for about 5 minutes until the onion is soft.
2 Add the squash to the onion mixture and continue to steam fry, stirring occasionally, for about 5 minutes until the flavours have combined.
3 Add the stock, cover and leave to simmer for 15–20 minutes until the squash is soft. Transfer to a liquidizer and blend until smooth. Reheat before serving.

SWEET BEETROOT SLAW

Raw beetroot adds a fresh crunchiness to this flavour-filled, detoxifying salad.

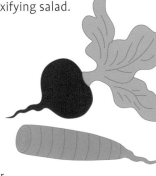

SERVES 3 AS A SIDE

★ 2 raw beetroot, peeled and grated
★ 2 carrots, peeled and grated
★ 1 sweet apple, peeled, cored and cut into thin slices
★ Juice 1 orange
★ 2 tbsp apple cider vinegar (with mother)

1 Mix all the ingredients together in the orange juice and vinegar.
2 Divide onto 3 plates and serve at once.

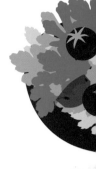

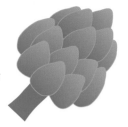

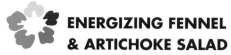 ## ENERGIZING FENNEL & ARTICHOKE SALAD

A traditional Mediterranean dish that promotes every youthing benefit.

SERVES 3 AS A SIDE

- ★ 1 lemon
- ★ 2 tbsp olive oil
- ★ 2 fennel bulbs

- ★ 1 small jar artichoke hearts, preserved in oil
- ★ 1 garlic clove, peeled and finely sliced
- ★ 1 tbsp chopped parsley

1 Squeeze the lemon juice into a bowl and add the olive oil.

2 Trim the fennel and remove any outer leaves. With a sharp knife cut the fennel bulb in half, and remove the hard middle core. Slice the flesh into very thin long shavings. Put the sliced fennel into the bowl with the lemon juice and olive oil.

3 Drain the artichokes and thinly slice. Add to the fennel with the garlic and parsley, toss in the dressing and serve at once.

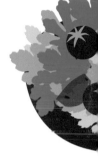

 ## ANTIOXIDANT-RICH POTATO SALAD

A filling lunch by itself! Radishes are great for the liver and high in testosterone, while the potato acts as a non-fattening carb.

SERVES 4

- ★ 500g new potatoes
- ★ Juice of 1 lemon
- ★ 1 avocado

- ★ 5 radishes, trimmed and thinly sliced
- ★ 2 tbsp olive oil
- ★ Small bunch watercress

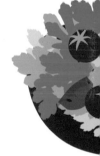

1 Put the potatoes in a saucepan and cover with water, bring to the boil and leave to simmer for about 15 minutes or until cooked. Drain and set aside to cool.

2 Put the lemon juice into a large bowl.

3 Halve the avocado, remove the stone and, using a spoon, scoop out the flesh and chop into cubes. Add to the lemon juice.

4 Cut the potatoes into cubes, then mix in with the avocado. Toss in the radishes, add the olive oil and stir to blend.

5 To serve, put the watercress on a plate and spoon over the potato salad.

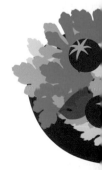

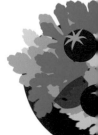

SPICED-UP BEANIE SALAD

Spicy and filling, this makes a swift, tasty, protein-packed lunch.

MAKES 2 GENEROUS PORTIONS

★ 240g tin kidney beans
★ 1 tbsp olive oil
★ 2 tbsp apple cider vinegar (with mother)
★ Juice of ½ lemon
★ ½ red onion, peeled and finely diced
★ ¼ red pepper, finely diced

★ ¼ green pepper, finely diced
★ 1 tsp de-seeded and chopped red chilli
★ 1 celery stick, trimmed and finely diced
★ 1 tbsp chopped coriander
★ 1 tbsp chopped parsley

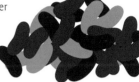

1 Rinse and drain the kidney beans.
2 Mix the oil, vinegar and lemon juice in a bowl, add the other ingredients and serve.

 ## SUPER SOBA NOODLE SALAD

An elegant salad with a hot and tangy bite.

SERVES 4

★ 140g soba noodles (buckwheat)
★ 200g soya beans, fresh or frozen
★ ½ mango, peeled, cored and cut into strips
★ 4 spring onions, trimmed and chopped
★ ½ chilli, de-seeded and finely sliced
★ Small bunch coriander, chopped
★ 300g beansprouts
★ 1 tbsp sesame seeds

FOR THE DRESSING
★ 2 tbsp sesame oil
★ 2 tbsp orange juice
★ 1 tsp lemon juice
★ 1 tsp lime juice
★ 2 tbsp apple cider vinegar (with mother)

1 Bring 1 litre water to the boil, then stir in the noodles. Reduce the heat and simmer for 5–7 minutes. Drain and rinse in cold water to stop the cooking process.
2 Bring a small pan of water to the boil and add the soya beans: cook for 1 minute at the boil then drain and rinse in cold water. Put in a large bowl with the noodles and remaining ingredients, except for the sesame seeds.
3 Mix the dressing ingredients together, then pour over the noodle salad, tossing well. Sprinkle over the sesame seeds and serve.

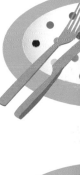
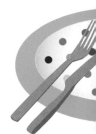

Main courses

Deliciously filling, nutritionally based main meals that are easy to cook and make you feel fantastic.

 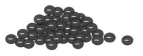

YOUTH-BOOST BURGER WITH SWEET TOMATO RELISH

The relish makes these beanie burgers come alive! Tamarind is traditionally used in the East to help with weight loss, digestion and as a detoxer.

SERVES 2

FOR THE BURGER
- ★ 200g kidney beans or aduki beans (tinned or dried)
- ★ 2 tbsp cashew nuts
- ★ 2 garlic cloves, peeled
- ★ 1 shallot, peeled
- ★ ½ carrot, peeled and grated
- ★ ½ tsp cumin
- ★ ½ tsp coriander
- ★ ½ tsp chilli powder (red)
- ★ 1 tsp tamarind paste, chopped
- ★ Spelt or non-wheat flour to coat
- ★ ½ tsp coconut oil

FOR THE TOMATO RELISH
- ★ ½ tsp coconut oil
- ★ 1 garlic clove, peeled and finely diced
- ★ 1 banana shallot, peeled and finely diced
- ★ ¼ tsp red (mild) chilli powder
- ★ 2 tomatoes, peeled (see page 101) and roughly chopped
- ★ 2 tbsp apple cider vinegar (with mother)
- ★ 1 tbsp tamarind paste

1 Preheat the grill to hot. If using tinned beans, rinse and drain them (if using dried, see page 101). Put the beans in a processor with the cashew nuts, garlic, shallot, carrot, spices and tamarind paste. Blend them as chunky or smooth as you like.

2 On a floured surface, divide the mixture into 2 and roll then flatten the top and sides to a burger shape. Heat the oil in a frying pan over a medium heat. Add the burgers with 4–6 tbsp water and steam fry (see page 100) for 1 minute to seal them. Then grill for 4–8 minutes on each side, or until they are done to your liking. They can be eaten raw, so don't worry about undercooking, it is all a question of taste.

3 To make the tomato relish, heat the oil in a saucepan over a gentle heat. Add the garlic, shallot and chilli powder with 4–6 tbsp water and steam fry until soft.

4 Add the tomatoes and stir to combine, then add the vinegar, tamarind and 3 tbsp water. Let the mixture reduce on a gentle heat until the tomatoes become a jam consistency. Serve hot or cold, with the burger.

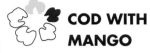 ## COD WITH MANGO

This packs a huge anti-ageing punch, with nutrient-rich avocados to rejuvenate skin.

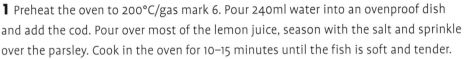

SERVES 4

- ★ 4 fillets of cod (around 120g each)
- ★ Juice of 2½ lemons
- ★ Himalayan salt with herbs
- ★ Small handful parsley, chopped
- ★ 2 avocados, peeled and stoned
- ★ ½ green chilli, chopped
- ★ Small handful basil
- ★ Small handful coriander
- ★ 1 mango, peeled and sliced into small squares

1 Preheat the oven to 200°C/gas mark 6. Pour 240ml water into an ovenproof dish and add the cod. Pour over most of the lemon juice, season with the salt and sprinkle over the parsley. Cook in the oven for 10–15 minutes until the fish is soft and tender.
2 Meanwhile, whiz the remaining ingredients, except the mango, in a liquidizer to a smooth paste. When the fish is ready, place on a serving platter in fillets or cut into chunky slices. Pour the puréed avocado mixture over, and garnish with the mango.

 ## GOAT'S CHEESE, AUBERGINE & BUTTER BEAN BAKE

Use a tangy goat's cheese to add extra flavour to the butter beans.

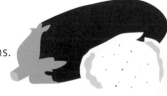

SERVES 3

- ★ ¼ tsp coconut oil
- ★ ½ onion, peeled and diced
- ★ 2 garlic cloves, peeled and diced
- ★ ½ aubergine, cut into small cubes
- ★ 100g Quick Tomato Sauce (see page 143)
- ★ 2 handfuls baby leaf spinach
- ★ 2 tbsp mixed chopped parsley and thyme
- ★ A few drops liquid aminos
- ★ 2 tbsp goat's cheese, diced or mashed
- ★ 240g tin butter beans, rinsed and drained
- ★ 3 tbsp pine nuts
- ★ 2 tbsp 'Cheese' Sprinkle (see page 144)

1 Preheat the oven to 160°C/gas mark 3. Heat the oil in a saucepan over a gentle heat. Add the onion and garlic with 4–6 tbsp water and steam fry (see page 100) for a few minutes until soft. Add the aubergine and a few tbsp water and cook for about 10 minutes. Add the remaining ingredients, except the pine nuts and 'cheese' sprinkle.
2 Take off the heat, mix and put in a small ovenproof dish. Sprinkle the pine nuts over the top and bake for about 20 minutes, until golden.

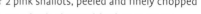

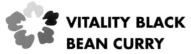 ## VITALITY BLACK BEAN CURRY

A hearty dish that's full of protein and ticks all the youthing boxes. Serve with rice or as a filling with baked potatoes.

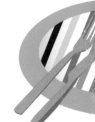

SERVES 4

- ★ 500ml homemade Vegetable Stock (see page 142)
- ★ 2 carrots, peeled and cubed
- ★ 2 parsnips, peeled and cubed
- ★ 420g tinned aduki beans/black beans, rinsed and drained
- ★ ½ tsp cumin seeds
- ★ ½ tsp fennel seeds
- ★ ½ tsp coconut oil
- ★ 2 pink shallots, peeled and finely chopped
- ★ 1 tsp finely chopped fresh root ginger
- ★ 3 garlic cloves, peeled and finely chopped
- ★ 250g tomatoes, peeled (see page 101) and roughly chopped
- ★ 1 tsp turmeric
- ★ 1 tsp garam masala
- ★ 1 tbsp lime juice
- ★ 1 tbsp chopped coriander

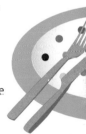

1 Pour the Vegetable Stock into a saucepan and bring to the boil on a high heat. Then add the carrots and parsnips, reduce the heat and let the vegetables simmer for about 5 minutes or until al dente. Stir in the beans and cook for a further 2 minutes at a simmer. Drain into a colander and reserve the bean mixture and liquid.

2 Heat a medium-sized frying pan for about 5 minutes (it should not be smoking), then dry-fry the cumin and fennel seeds for about 1 minute, stirring, until they release a fragrant smell. Reserve the seeds.

3 Heat the oil in a heavy-based deep frying pan or saucepan on a medium heat. Add the shallots with 4–6 tbsp water and steam fry (see page 100) for about 5 minutes until translucent. Stir in the seeds, ginger and garlic and cook for a further 30 seconds.

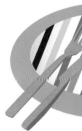

4 Add the tomatoes and 100ml of the reserved stock. Keep on a low heat, stirring from time to time, until the tomatoes start to disintegrate – about 2 minutes.

5 Stir in the turmeric and continue cooking for 2 minutes more – add more of the reserved stock if the mixture looks dry. Take off the heat.

6 Add the bean mixture to the spicy tomato mixture and stir to blend. Simmer together for 5–8 minutes on a very low heat, adding more stock if the curry looks dry.

7 At the last minute add the garam masala, lime juice and coriander. Serve at once.

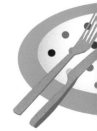

TRAD THAI CURRY WITH BARLEY

Substituting barley for rice gives this green veg curry a nutty chewiness – and helps raise its youthing potential.

SERVES 2

★ 150g pearl barley

FOR THE GREEN THAI PASTE
★ ½ green chilli, de-seeded and chopped
★ 5cm fresh root ginger, peeled and chopped
★ 4 spring onions, trimmed and chopped
★ 3 kaffir lime leaves, roughly torn
★ 2 sticks lemongrass, chopped
★ 1 tsp turmeric
★ 400ml can coconut milk

FOR THE CURRY
★ 1 onion, peeled and chopped
★ 1 tsp coconut oil
★ ½ aubergine, cubed
★ 1 sweet potato, peeled and cubed
★ 6 kaffir lime leaves
★ 2 tbsp chopped coriander
★ 30g cashew nuts, chopped
★ Squeeze of lime juice

1 Put the barley in 500ml water, bring to the boil and cook for 20–25 minutes.
2 To make the Thai paste, put all the ingredients into a liquidizer together with 2 tbsp of the coconut milk. Blend to form a paste.
3 To make the curry, sauté the onion in the oil in a large pan for 2–3 minutes, until soft and translucent. Add the aubergine and sweet potato and sauté for a further 3–5 minutes until soft but not falling apart. Add the Thai paste and cook for 2 minutes.
4 Add the rest of the coconut milk and the 6 kaffir lime leaves. Cook for a further 10 minutes. Once the vegetables are soft add the coriander and cashew nuts.
5 Drain the barley. Before serving, add a squeeze of lime juice to the curry. Serve on top of the barley.

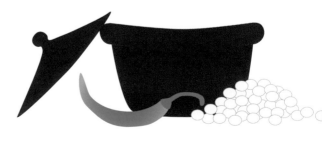

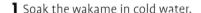

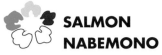

SALMON NABEMONO

A traditional one-pot Japanese dish with many variations – you can use pak choi, Savoy cabbage, watercress, mangetout, spinach .... If you add tofu or eggs put them in at the last minute. Serve with rice or udon noodles on the side.

SERVES 2

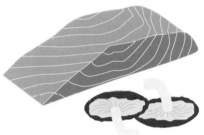

- ★ 50g wakame seaweed
- ★ 120g shiitake mushrooms, sliced
- ★ 2 tsp liquid aminos
- ★ 2 tsp apple cider vinegar (with mother)
- ★ 2 carrots, peeled and cut into 1cm cubes
- ★ 2 potatoes, peeled and cut into 1cm cubes
- ★ 1 parsnip, peeled and cut into 1cm cubes
- ★ 50g water chestnuts, sliced
- ★ 340g fillet skinned salmon
- ★ 50g beansprouts
- ★ 3 spring onions, trimmed and finely chopped

1 Soak the wakame in cold water.

2 To make a broth, put the mushrooms in a pan with the liquid aminos, vinegar and 500ml water and simmer gently for 10 minutes.

3 Add the carrots, potatoes, parsnip and water chestnuts and simmer gently for a further 10 minutes.

4 Just before the vegetables are cooked, drain the wakame, then add to the broth with the whole piece of salmon (keep it whole while cooking) and the beansprouts. Bring back to a gentle simmer for a few minutes.

5 Just before serving, add the spring onions, take the pan off the heat and serve in the pan on the table with the salmon cut in half.

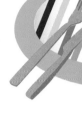

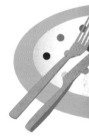

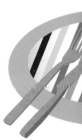

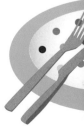

SUPER YOUTHING STROGANOFF

Root veg and kidney beans give a flavoursome dish high in youthing antioxidants.

SERVES 4

- ★ ¼ tsp coconut oil
- ★ ½ onion, peeled and finely chopped
- ★ 1 garlic clove, peeled and finely chopped
- ★ 170g butternut squash, peeled and diced
- ★ 1 carrot, peeled and diced
- ★ 110g celeriac, peeled and diced
- ★ 100g shiitake mushrooms, thinly sliced

- ★ ½ tsp paprika
- ★ ¼ tsp nutmeg
- ★ 200ml homemade Vegetable Stock (see page 142)
- ★ 240g tin kidney beans, rinsed and drained
- ★ 2 tbsp goat's yoghurt
- ★ A few drops liquid aminos
- ★ 1 tbsp chopped parsley

1 Heat the oil in a saucepan over a gentle heat. Add the onion and garlic with 4–6 tbsp water and steam fry (see page 100) for a few minutes until soft. Add the vegetables to the onion and garlic and continue to steam fry for a few minutes more.
2 Stir in the paprika and nutmeg and continue cooking for a few minutes. Then add the stock, cover and leave to simmer over a gentle heat for about 10 minutes. Add the beans and cook for another couple of minutes until the vegetables are soft.
3 Remove from the heat and stir in the yoghurt, liquid aminos and chopped parsley, and serve with steamed rice.

SPINACH-STUFFED SALMON

Both salmon and walnuts are rich in soothing, anti-inflammatory omega–3s. You can also serve this dish without the rice, if you don't want to have carbs late at night.

SERVES 4

- ★ 140g brown rice
- ★ ½ tsp coconut oil
- ★ 1 small onion, peeled and chopped
- ★ 2 garlic cloves, peeled and chopped
- ★ 1 tbsp chopped tarragon
- ★ 240g spinach

- ★ 125g walnuts, chopped
- ★ Grated zest of 1 lemon
- ★ 700g salmon fillet
- ★ Lemon juice
- ★ Freshly ground black pepper

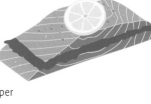

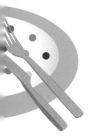

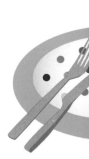

1 Cook the rice, using double the amount of water as rice – it will take about 25 minutes. To stop rice going mushy, put a lid on the pan and allow to stand for the last 10 minutes of the cooking time, rather than simmering it dry.

2 Meanwhile, preheat the oven to 200°C/gas mark 6.

3 Heat the oil in a saucepan over a gentle heat. Add the onion with 4–6 tbsp water and steam fry (see page 100) for a few minutes until soft. Add the garlic and tarragon and cook for a few seconds before adding the spinach. Stir until it has wilted, then add the walnuts and lemon zest. Stir for a few minutes and take off the heat.

4 Drain the rice and, once it has cooled slightly, stir into the spinach/walnut mix.

5 Cut the salmon into 4 portions. Slice each piece of salmon through the middle and put the spinach/rice mix in between the 2 slices of salmon, season with lemon juice and pepper. Hold together with a cocktail stick, then put in the oven and cook for 15 minutes until the fish is cooked through.

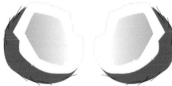

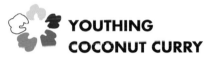 ## YOUTHING COCONUT CURRY

Eat with brown/black rice, and a cucumber, mint and yoghurt raita. Or just on its own.

SERVES 4

- ★ ¾ tsp turmeric
- ★ ¾ tsp chilli powder
- ★ ¾ tsp ground ginger
- ★ 1 tbsp mango juice
- ★ 1 tsp chopped tamarind
- ★ 1 tsp coconut oil
- ★ 1 tsp black mustard seeds
- ★ 2 tsp cumin seeds
- ★ 1 garlic clove, peeled and chopped
- ★ 1 small onion, peeled and thinly sliced longways
- ★ 1 tsp finely chopped fresh root ginger
- ★ 800ml (2 tins) coconut milk
- ★ 160g butternut squash, peeled and cubed
- ★ 1 potato, peeled and cut into 1cm cubes
- ★ 1 parsnip, peeled and cut into 1cm cubes
- ★ 150g cauliflower, broken into florets
- ★ 2 tbsp chopped coriander, to serve
- ★ 50g cashew nuts, toasted, to serve

1 Put the spices, mango juice and tamarind into a food processor and blend until smooth. Then heat the oil in a saucepan until hot. Add the black mustard and cumin seeds and cook until they start to pop. Add the garlic, onion and ginger and sauté for about 5 minutes until the onion is soft.

2 Add the turmeric paste and cook for about a minute until it becomes fragrant. Stir in the coconut milk and add the vegetables. Simmer for 20–30 minutes, stirring occasionally, until the vegetables are al dente. To serve, stir in the coriander and sprinkle over the cashew nuts.

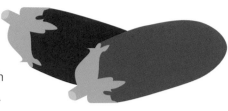

ANTIOXIDANT AUBERGINES

With garlic and shiitake mushrooms, this recipe is rich in antioxidants, iron and immune-boosting nutrients.

SERVES 1 AS A MAIN DISH OR MAKES SIDE DISHES FOR 2

- ★ 2 aubergines
- ★ ½ tsp coconut oil
- ★ 1 onion, peeled and finely chopped
- ★ 2 garlic cloves, peeled and finely chopped
- ★ 3 shiitake mushrooms, finely chopped
- ★ 2 tsp dried paprika
- ★ 2 tsp dried oregano
- ★ 2 tsp fresh thyme
- ★ 20g pine nuts
- ★ 1 tsp lemon juice

1 Split both aubergines lengthways, score the flesh in a criss-cross pattern with a knife and bake for 20–30 minutes at 180°C/gas mark 4 until softened.

2 Meanwhile, heat the oil and steam fry (see page 100) the onion and garlic until soft. Add the mushrooms, fry a little more until soft – you may need to add more water to help soften and fry the onion more evenly.

3 Take the aubergines out of the oven and remove the flesh by scooping out with a spoon. You can be quite rough as you need only two halves (so will be throwing two skins away).

4 Add the aubergine flesh to the onion mixture and stir in the paprika, oregano, thyme and pine nuts. Heat through, then at the last minute add the lemon juice.

5 Stuff the skins of the aubergine with the mixture, then serve.

BAKED POTATO WITH WASABI

So simple and delicious. Soothing on the tummy as well as satisfying as a meal. Eat with a green salad.

SERVES 1

- ★ 250g baking potato
- ★ ½ tsp wasabi paste (made up from wasabi powder)
- ★ 1 tsp goat's cheese
- ★ 2 tsp olive oil
- ★ 1 tsp chopped parsley
- ★ ¼ medium hot chilli, chopped (optional)

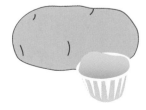

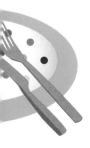

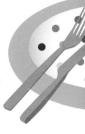

1 Preheat the oven to 200°C/gas mark 6.

2 Put the potato on a shelf in the oven and bake for about an hour until cooked.

3 Remove from the oven, cut the potato in half and scoop out the flesh leaving the skins intact.

4 Mash the wasabi paste, goat's cheese, olive oil, parsley and chilli (if using) together with the potato flesh. Spoon the potato/wasabi mix back into the potato skins and return to the oven for 10 minutes. When the potato is brown on top, it's ready.

 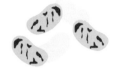

BORLOTTI BEAN & CAVOLO NERO CASSEROLE

A light and tasty youth booster. Cavolo nero is high in antioxidants, calcium and phytonutrients.

SERVES 4

- ★ ½ tsp coconut oil
- ★ 1 red onion, peeled and diced
- ★ 4 garlic cloves, peeled and finely chopped
- ★ 2 celery sticks, trimmed and chopped
- ★ 2 carrots, peeled and cubed
- ★ 160g celeriac, peeled and cubed
- ★ 2 tbsp chopped flat-leaf parsley
- ★ 2 tomatoes, peeled (see page 101) and roughly chopped

- ★ 2kg cavolo nero (or Swiss chard, Savoy cabbage or kale)
- ★ 500g tinned borlotti or butter beans, rinsed and drained
- ★ 700ml homemade Vegetable Stock (see page 142) or use water
- ★ Freshly ground black pepper
- ★ Olive oil, to drizzle

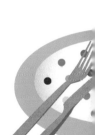

1 Heat the oil in a saucepan over a medium heat. Add the onion, garlic, celery, carrots, celeriac and parsley with 4–6 tbsp water and steam fry (see page 100) for about 15 minutes until the vegetables are al dente.

2 Add the tomatoes and cook on a gentle heat for another 15 minutes.

3 Meanwhile, de-stalk the cavolo nero and coarsely chop the leaves. (If using other brassicas, make sure the outer leaves and hard stems are removed.) Add the cavolo nero and 300g of the beans to the vegetable mix. Cover with the Vegetable Stock (you may not use all of it or you may need to add water) and leave for 30 minutes.

4 In a food processor, purée the remaining beans with about 1 tbsp water. Add the purée to the bean/vegetable mixture and stir to combine. If you need more liquid, add Vegetable Stock or water – it should be a soupy consistency.

5 Before serving, season with ground black pepper and drizzle with olive oil.

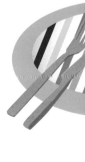

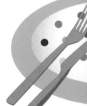

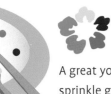 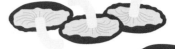 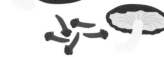

MUSHROOM BARLEY RISOTTO

A great youth booster. For more protein and extra flavour, sprinkle goat/sheep's cheese on top.

SERVES 4

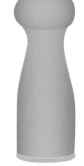

- ★ 10g dried or 4 fresh, medium-sized shiitake mushrooms, sliced
- ★ ½ tsp coconut oil
- ★ 1 small onion, peeled and chopped
- ★ 2 garlic cloves, peeled and chopped
- ★ 100g pearl barley
- ★ 600ml homemade Vegetable Stock (see page 142) or mushroom juice (or just veg stock if using fresh mushrooms)

- ★ ½ tbsp chopped parsley
- ★ ½ tbsp chopped coriander
- ★ ½ tsp liquid aminos
- ★ Black pepper

1 If using dried mushrooms, soak them in boiling water for 30 minutes, then drain, saving the liquid for use as part of the stock.

2 In a medium-sized pan, heat the oil and steam fry (see page 100) the onion and garlic on a gentle heat for about 5 minutes until soft. Add the mushrooms (if fresh) and sauté for another 5 minutes.

3 When the onion is translucent, add the barley (if using dried mushrooms add them now) and stir until coated in oil.

4 Keep the stock warm in a small pan. Add 4 ladles of hot stock to the barley, to cover. Simmer until the barley has absorbed nearly all the liquid, stirring frequently. Add more stock in small amounts until absorbed, keep stirring, and continue in this way until the barley is cooked (about 20 minutes) though still al dente. It should look slightly wet and creamy, but not like a soup.

5 At the last moment, stir in the parsley, coriander, liquid aminos and pepper to taste. Serve at once.

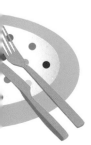

Side dishes

These vegetable dishes go well with the main courses or as light meals on their own with baked potatoes, rice or bread.

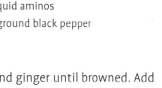

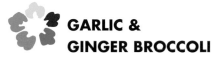

GARLIC & GINGER BROCCOLI

Simple and tasty, this ticks all the youthing boxes.

SERVES 2

* ★ 1 tbsp coconut oil
* ★ 3 garlic cloves, peeled and chopped
* ★ 60g fresh root ginger, peeled and chopped
* ★ 1 head of broccoli, broken into florets
* ★ ½ tsp liquid aminos
* ★ Freshly ground black pepper

1 Heat the oil in a large frying pan and fry the garlic and ginger until browned. Add 120ml water and the broccoli and poach for a few minutes until the broccoli is soft.
2 Add the liquid aminos and black pepper to taste.

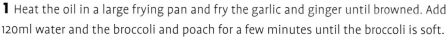

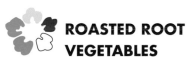

ROASTED ROOT VEGETABLES

A tasty dish that you can serve hot as a side, or cold as a salad on a bed of rocket.

SERVES 2

* ★ 200g butternut squash
* ★ 1 beetroot
* ★ ½ sweet potato
* ★ 1 carrot
* ★ 170g celeriac
* ★ ½ red onion, peeled
* ★ 4 garlic cloves, peeled
* ★ 1 tsp chopped thyme
* ★ 1 tbsp pine nuts
* ★ 2 tbsp pumpkin seeds

1 Preheat the oven to 200°C/gas mark 6.
2 Peel and cut the butternut squash, beetroot, sweet potato, carrot and celeriac into 2cm chunks. Cut the onion into 8 slices, and slice the garlic into thin slithers.
3 Place all the veggies on a baking tray with the garlic slithers and fresh thyme, and roast for about 15 minutes until cooked. Lightly toast the pine nuts and pumpkin seeds until they turn brown, then sprinkle over the vegetables and serve.

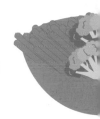

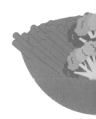

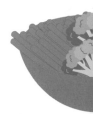

STUFFED COURGETTES

Serve topped with the Quick Tomato Sauce (see page 143) as a starter or side dish.

MAKES 2 STARTERS OR A SIDE DISH FOR 4

- ★ 2 courgettes
- ★ ½ tsp coconut oil
- ★ 2 garlic cloves, peeled and chopped
- ★ 2 small shallots, peeled and diced

- ★ 2 tsp finely chopped thyme
- ★ 1 tsp finely chopped parsley
- ★ 2 tsp nutritional yeast
- ★ 1 tsp finely chopped pine nuts

1 Preheat the oven to 160°C/gas mark 3.

2 Trim the top and bottom of each courgette, then divide each one along its length into three equal-sized pieces. Using a melon baller, scoop the flesh from the courgettes, leaving six bases for the herb stuffing. Roughly chop the flesh.

3 Heat the oil in a saucepan over a gentle heat. Add the onion and shallots with 4–6 tbsp water and steam fry (see page 100) for a few minutes until soft. Add the courgette flesh and continue to steam fry for about 10 minutes until the courgettes break down. Add the thyme and parsley and cook for 5 minutes more or until the courgettes are tender. Remove from the heat and stir in the yeast and pine nuts.

4 Place the 6 courgette skins on a baking tray and fill with the courgette pine nut mix. Cook for 30–40 minutes until the skin is nice and soft. You can add some water to the baking tray to keep the courgettes moist while cooking.

5 Take out and serve at once with 2 tbsp Tomato Sauce on top.

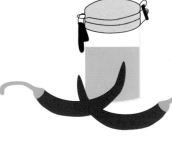

SOOTHING COCONUT DHAL

Yummy with steamed fish, rice or baked potato.

SERVES 2

- ★ 200g yellow split peas
- ★ ½ tsp ground cumin
- ★ ½ tsp turmeric
- ★ 1 tin (400ml) coconut milk
- ★ 2 medium-hot chillies, de-seeded and chopped
- ★ ½ tsp coconut oil

- ★ 1 heaped tsp black onion seeds
- ★ 6 curry leaves
- ★ 3 shallots, peeled and finely chopped
- ★ 3 garlic cloves, peeled and chopped
- ★ 2 tomatoes, peeled (see page 101) and cut into eighths
- ★ 2 tbsp chopped coriander

1 Rinse the split peas in a sieve under a cold tap. Drain. Place them in a saucepan, and add the cumin, turmeric, coconut milk and 500ml water. Bring to the boil, put the lid on the pan with a little gap for the steam to escape, and simmer for 30–40 minutes, stirring occasionally.

2 Add the chillies and some more water (up to another 200ml) if the dhal seems overly thick. Simmer for another 15 minutes.

3 Meanwhile, heat the oil in a frying pan over a medium heat and brown the onion seeds and curry leaves. Add the shallots and garlic together with 4–6 tbsp water and steam fry (see page 100) until they start to colour. Stir frequently.

4 Add the tomatoes, cook until soft but not collapsed (they need to hold their shape).

5 Stir the tomato mixture into the dhal, add the coriander and serve at once.

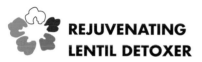 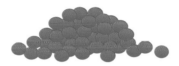

REJUVENATING LENTIL DETOXER

This is a rich, flavoursome lentil dish that goes extremely well with fish, grilled vegetables or beanie burgers.

SERVES 4

- ★ 200g Puy lentils, rinsed
- ★ ½ onion, peeled and chopped in half
- ★ 1 carrot, peeled and quartered
- ★ 1 red chilli, halved and de-seeded
- ★ 3 garlic cloves, peeled and left whole
- ★ 2 bay leaves
- ★ 2–3cm fresh root ginger, peeled and sliced into chunks
- ★ 5 parsley stalks or a sprig of thyme
- ★ 1 tbsp chopped coriander
- ★ Homemade Vegetable Stock (see page 142) or water to cover

FOR THE SAUCE
- ★ 2 tbsp apple cider vinegar (with mother)
- ★ 3 tbsp olive oil
- ★ Freshly ground black pepper
- ★ Few drops liquid aminos

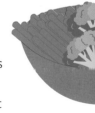

1 Put the lentils in a deep saucepan. Add the rest of the vegetables, herbs and spices and then pour over enough Vegetable Stock or water to cover. Bring to the boil then reduce the heat and leave to simmer for about 20 minutes. The lentils should be soft but still have a bite.

2 Remove the lentils from the heat and drain. Remove the carrot, onion, ginger, bay leaves and parsley stalks (or thyme), leaving only the garlic and chilli behind.

3 While the lentils are still warm, add the vinegar, olive oil, black pepper and a few drops of liquid aminos to taste.

ASIAN CRUNCHY STIR-FRY

Serve as a side with fish or curry, or eat raw as a salad (leave out the the ginger and garlic) with a sesame seed oil and apple cider vinegar dressing.

SERVES 6

- ★ 2 whole pak choi
- ★ 2 carrots
- ★ ½ green and ½ red pepper
- ★ 4 spring onions, trimmed and finely chopped
- ★ 2cm fresh root ginger, finely diced
- ★ 4 garlic cloves, peeled and finely diced
- ★ ½ red chilli, de-seeded and finely diced
- ★ 200g beansprouts
- ★ ½ tsp coconut oil
- ★ 2 tbsp mixed finely chopped coriander and mint
- ★ Few drops liquid aminos
- ★ Juice of 1 lime
- ★ 1 tsp apple cider vinegar (with mother)

1 Wash and cut the pak choi into 2cm strips including the green leafy part. Peel and cut the carrots into long thin matchsticks. De-seed the peppers and cut as the carrots.

2 Mix together the chopped veg with the ginger, garlic, chilli and beansprouts.

3 Heat a wok or large frying pan over a medium heat for several minutes. Add the oil and swirl around to coat the pan. Once hot (but not smoking), add the veg mix and stir-fry, stirring for several minutes. Remove from the heat while the veg are still crunchy.

4 Stir in the chopped herbs, liquid aminos, lime juice and vinegar, and serve at once.

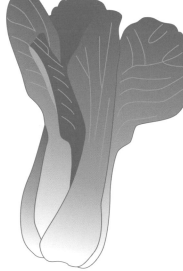

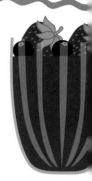
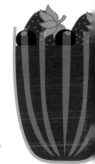
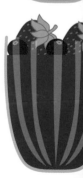

Puddings

There are lots to choose from here and in the detox section (see pages 83–5). None of them have added sugar, honey or other sweeteners. Don't feel you have to eat one a day: instead, start thinking of puddings as a treat to be eaten perhaps two or three times a week, when you have people round for supper, or when you are genuinely hungry after a meal. You can also eat these puddings as snacks or for breakfast · having your sugar fix early in the day is better than eating it after 7.30pm.

CREAMY COCONUT & PINEAPPLE BLACK RICE PUD

This no-added sugar rice pudding manages to taste deliciously sweet because of the pineapple and coconut. Black rice is full of iron and fibre, a slow-release carb that has the nutritional edge over brown rice – it is expensive, though, so mix It half and half with brown rice if you like.

SERVES 4

- ★ 200g black rice (or organic brown rice)
- ★ 250ml pineapple juice (fresh if possible)
- ★ 250ml coconut milk
- ★ 1 stick cinnamon or ½ tsp ground cinnamon
- ★ 5 cardamom pods, crushed
- ★ ½ stick lemongrass (optional)

TO DECORATE
- ★ Fresh pineapple chunks
- ★ Handful toasted almonds
- ★ Mint leaves

1 Soak the rice, preferably overnight or for 2 hours, in cold water to soften. Drain.
2 Put the rice, juice and coconut milk with 200ml water in a heavy-based pan. Bring to a simmer, then add the spices and cook, stirring regularly, for about 30 minutes. If you like the rice softer, cook for a further 10 minutes. If the liquid evaporates too quickly, add a little more water as needed.
3 When the rice is cooked and the milk has thickened, turn off the heat. Remove the cinnamon stick, cardamom and lemongrass (if using).
4 Serve in bowls, decorated with pineapple, toasted almonds and mint.

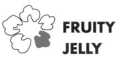 **FRUITY
JELLY**

Jelly is something of a forgotten classic – this tasty, youthing version is sugar and gelatine free. Serve with custard or ice cream.

SERVES 2

★ 200ml freshly squeezed orange juice
★ 1 tsp agar flakes
★ Fruit of your choice, chopped small

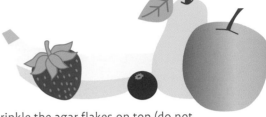

1 Place the orange juice in a saucepan and sprinkle the agar flakes on top (do not stir). Bring the mixture to the boil and simmer for 2–3 minutes.
2 Take off the heat and add the desired chopped fresh fruit. Pour into 2 bowls and put in the fridge to set.

**BLUEBERRY LAYERED COULIS
WITH A CHILLI KICK**

Banana and yoghurt are soothing for the gut, while blueberries contain exceptionally youthing bioflavonoids, thought to be helpful for improving learning, vision and some age-related conditions.

SERVES 2

★ 1–2 bananas
★ Pinch of chilli flakes
★ Juice of ½ lime

★ 200g blueberries
★ 200g goat/sheep's milk yoghurt

1 Mash the banana in a pestle and mortar, add a pinch of chilli flakes (to suit your taste) and the lime juice and mix well.
2 Put the blueberries into a liquidizer (reserve 2 for decoration) and whiz for a minute. Then strain the mixture through a sieve into a bowl.
3 Place a layer of banana mush at the bottom of 2 tall glasses, spoon some blueberry coulis on top, then add a thick topping of yoghurt. Decorate with a blueberry.

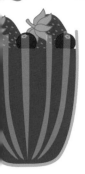
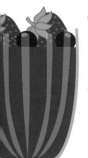

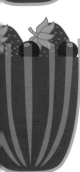

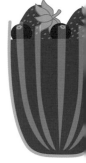
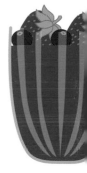
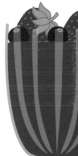
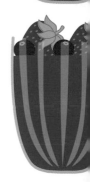
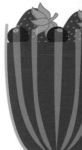

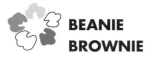

BEANIE BROWNIE

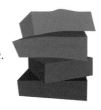

These sugar-free brownies are rich in antioxidants and taste deliciously chocolatey! They will keep for several days in the fridge.

MAKES 12

- ★ 100g dark chocolate (at least 70% cocoa solids)
- ★ 80g coconut oil
- ★ 30g cocoa powder
- ★ 100g tinned aduki beans
- ★ 100g Medjool dates, chopped
- ★ 50ml coconut milk
- ★ 45g ground almonds
- ★ 1 egg
- ★ 2 tsp vanilla extract

1 Grease and line a 20 x 10 x 6cm loaf tin. Preheat the oven to 180°C/gas mark 4.

2 Melt the chocolate and coconut oil in a pan over a very low heat. Stir in the cocoa and remove from the heat.

3 Rinse and drain the aduki beans, then put into a liquidizer with the dates, coconut milk and ground almonds and pulse to form a thick paste.

4 In a large separate bowl, beat the egg and vanilla extract together.

5 Fold the bean mixture into the chocolate, then add to the egg. Pour the batter into the tin and bake for 25–30 minutes (don't overcook, brownies are best a little gooey).

6 Leave to cool, and chill before serving.

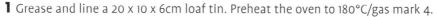

VANILLA SOYA CUSTARD

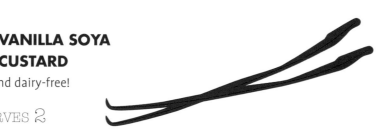

Delicious and dairy-free!

SERVES 2

- ★ ½ vanilla pod
- ★ 200ml soya milk
- ★ 1 heaped tsp potato flour
- ★ 1 tbsp Sweet Apricot Paste (see page 145)

1 Split the vanilla pod down the centre and scrape out the vanilla seeds.

2 Put the soya milk, vanilla seeds and pod into a small saucepan, and heat gently.

3 Put the potato flour into a small bowl and, once the milk is heated, pour it over the potato flour, stirring continuously until smooth. Put the custard back into the saucepan and heat gently, stirring until the custard begins to thicken. Remove the vanilla pod. To serve, stir in the Sweet Apricot Paste, according to taste.

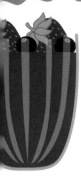

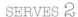

YOUTHING SUMMER PUDDING

An antioxidant-rich, sugar-free version of a traditional British pud, delicious with sheep's yoghurt or ice cream.

SERVES 2

★ ¾ of a white gluten-free bread loaf

FOR THE SAUCE
★ 8 large strawberries
★ 200g raspberries

FOR THE FILLING
★ 100g strawberries, topped and sliced
★ 150g blueberries
★ 150g raspberries
★ A squeeze of lemon juice

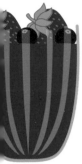

1 To make the sauce, put the berries into a liquidizer with 60ml water, and whiz until liquid. If the sauce looks too thick, thin it down by adding a bit more water – you want a runny consistency that will easily seep into the bread.

2 Cut the bread into 1cm thick slices, removing the crusts.

3 Infuse a few slices of bread with the liquefied fruit mixture and use to line the base and sides of a 600ml pudding basin or Pyrex bowl.

4 To make the filling, put 1 tbsp of each of the three fruits into the basin or bowl, sprinkling a few drops of lemon juice on top.

5 Dip some more of the bread into the sauce and entirely cover the fruit in the basin or bowl with the soaked bread. Then add more fruit and lemon juice, repeating the process until the basin is filled. The final layer should be the soaked bread at the top of the basin. Keep any reserved juice in the fridge.

6 Cover the pudding with greaseproof paper and put a plate on top that fits the basin or bowl exactly. Put something heavy on top of the plate to weigh it down. Leave in the fridge overnight.

7 Before serving, ease the pudding out of the basin or bowl by running a palette knife around the inside of the container. Then gently turn out on to a plate, spooning any reserved sauce over the pudding.

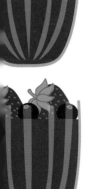

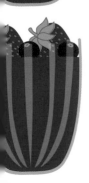

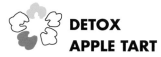 **DETOX APPLE TART**

Apples are good detoxers as they are high in pectin, which aids digestion. The tart will keep for 4–5 days in the fridge.

SERVES 4

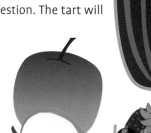

FOR THE PASTRY
- ★ 30g rice flour
- ★ 15g ground almonds
- ★ 1 tbsp tahini
- ★ ½ tbsp sunflower oil

FOR THE FILLING
- ★ 4 eating apples
- ★ 50g Medjool dates
- ★ 1 tsp ground cinnamon
- ★ 2 pears

1 Preheat the oven to 180°C/gas mark 4.

2 To make the pastry, put the rice flour, ground almonds, tahini and oil in a food processor. Pulse until the mixture becomes like breadcrumbs. Slowly add 150ml water and continue pulsing until the mixture comes together like a pastry ball.

3 Place the pastry in a 20cm round tart tin with removable base, pushing it into the sides to give an even layer. Bake in the oven for 10–15 minutes or until it starts to brown.

4 To make the filling, peel, core and chop the apples, and stone and roughly chop the dates. Put the apples, dates and cinnamon in a pan with 2 tbsp water. Stew on a gentle heat until the apples are soft – adding more water to the mixture if needed. Allow to cool for 10 minutes. Once cool, purée in a food processor and spread the filling onto the pastry.

5 Peel and core the pears. Finely slice them lengthways for the decoration, layering them evenly in a circular pattern around the tin. Sprinkle lemon juice on top.

6 Serve with custard or ice cream.

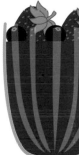
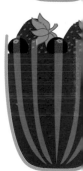
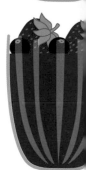
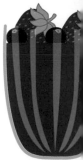

Snacks

It's always better to have a youthing snack to hand rather than buying something 'healthy' (inevitably full of fat and sugar). Try these:

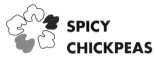 ## SPICY CHICKPEAS

A savoury snack nibble or add to salads and soups as croutons. Keeps for 2 weeks.

SERVES 4 AS A SNACK

- ★ 275g chickpeas, dried or tinned
- ★ 1 tsp paprika
- ★ ½ tsp turmeric
- ★ ½ tsp ground cumin
- ★ ½ tsp dried chilli flakes

- ★ 1 tbsp coconut or rice bran oil
- ★ ½ tsp liquid aminos
- ★ 3 garlic cloves, peeled and finely chopped
- ★ Squeeze of lemon

1 Preheat the oven to 200°C/gas mark 6.
2 If using dried chickpeas, see page 101. If using tinned chickpeas, rinse well, and pat dry with kitchen paper.
3 Mix the paprika, turmeric, cumin and chilli in a small bowl. Put to one side.
4 Mix the oil, liquid aminos, garlic and lemon juice together in another small bowl.
5 Roll the chickpeas in the liquid ingredients, then in the spicy mix.
6 Spread the chickpeas on a baking tray and cook in the oven for 40 minutes or until crunchy, moving them around from time to time so they are browned on all sides.

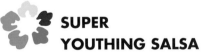 ## SUPER YOUTHING SALSA

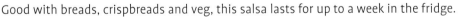

Good with breads, crispbreads and veg, this salsa lasts for up to a week in the fridge.

MAKES 1 BOWLFUL

- ★ 100g spinach
- ★ 2 garlic cloves, peeled
- ★ ¼ onion, peeled
- ★ 1 spicy chilli, de-seeded

- ★ 25g parsley sprigs
- ★ 50ml cold-pressed extra-virgin olive oil
- ★ 1 tsp apple cider vinegar (with mother)
- ★ Juice of 1 lemon

1 Put all the ingredients in a liquidizer and whiz until smooth.

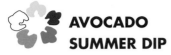 ## AVOCADO SUMMER DIP

Hot with a fresh, minty tang, this contains alkalizing cucumber and lemon.

SERVES 2 AS A SNACK

- ★ ¼ cucumber
- ★ ½ spring onion, trimmed
- ★ ½ avocado, peeled and stoned
- ★ 1 tbsp lemon juice, freshly squeezed
- ★ ¼ green chilli
- ★ 6 mint leaves
- ★ Handful basil
- ★ Handful parsley

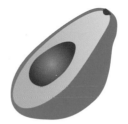

1 Put all the ingredients into a liquidizer and blend until smooth, thick and creamy.

2 Eat as a dip with raw vegetables or any of the breads on pages 138–9.

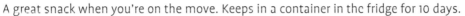

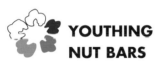 ## YOUTHING NUT BARS

A great snack when you're on the move. Keeps in a container in the fridge for 10 days.

MAKES 6 BARS

- ★ 110g jumbo rolled oats
- ★ 50g whole almonds, roughly chopped
- ★ 50g sesame seeds
- ★ 50g sunflower seeds
- ★ 50g pumpkin seeds
- ★ 220g Sweet Apricot Paste (see page 145)
- ★ 110g unsulphured apricots, blanched and chopped
- ★ 50g mixed almonds and sunflower seeds, ground together finely

FOR THE PASTE
- ★ 100g tahini

FOR THE CHOCOLATE TOPPING (OPTIONAL)
- ★ 100g dark chocolate (80% cocoa solids)

1 Preheat the oven to 180°C/gas mark 4. Put the oats, almonds and seeds on a baking tray and roast lightly in the oven for 10 minutes. Set aside for later.

2 Mix the tahini and apricot paste. Add the apricots and ground seed mix. Stir well.

3 Thoroughly mix together the warmed oats/seed mixture with the tahini mixture, then spread evenly in a 20cm square deep-sided cake tin. Cool in the fridge.

4 If you want a treat, you can add a chocolate topping to the bars. First melt the chocolate in a heatproof bowl set over a pan of simmering water. Then spread on top of the nut bar with a hot palette knife or the back of a spoon. Leave to set in the fridge and then chop into squares.

Breads and cakes

Most people eat bread every day but actually it's healthier to eat it just a few times a week and incorporate other forms of grain carbs into your diet. Still, bread is handy for breakfast and to accompany soups and salads. The bread recipes here are unusual, delicious and very youthing – no yeast, no sugar and no additives. The cake and scones are more-ish, so restraint might be needed!

PUMPKIN SEED & TOMATO BREAD

With a nutty, almost malty sweetness and rich tomato tang, this bread makes a special weekend or dinner party treat.

MAKES 1 MEDIUM LOAF OR 6 ROLLS

- ★ 150g buckwheat flour
- ★ 80g spelt flour
- ★ 1½ tsp baking powder
- ★ 1 tsp xanthum gum
- ★ 30g pumpkin seeds
- ★ 50ml goat's milk
- ★ 90ml tomato juice, freshly squeezed (about 1½ tomatoes)
- ★ 50ml goat's yoghurt
- ★ 1 egg
- ★ 3 large oven-dried tomatoes (see page 142), with their oil and finely chopped

1 Preheat the oven to 180°C/gas mark 4.

2 Mix the buckwheat and spelt flours in a bowl with the baking powder, xanthum gum and pumpkin seeds.

3 Put the goat's milk, tomato juice, yoghurt and egg in a separate mixing bowl and blend for 1 minute with a hand-held electric whisk on a medium/high speed until you can see bubbles on top of the liquid. If it is curdling, don't worry, it will come back when the flour is added.

4 Add the dried tomatoes to the flour mixture and stir until combined. Make a well in the middle and mix in the yoghurt/milk mixture.

5 Rub your hands lightly with a few drops of olive oil and knead for a minute or so until the dough is thick and handling well.

6 Pick up the dough and make it into a loaf shape, or break into round dough balls to make small rolls. Place on a baking tray and bake in the oven for 35–40 minutes until golden brown and sounding hollow when you tap the bottom.

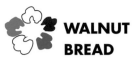

WALNUT BREAD

This nutty, dense bread is delicious toasted or plain and it will last for 4–5 days in your bread bin.

MAKES 1 SMALL LOAF

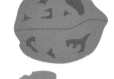
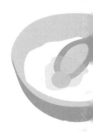

- ★ 40g walnuts
- ★ 70g kamut flour
- ★ 1 tsp potato flour (to help bind the bread)
- ★ 60g buckwheat flour
- ★ 1 tsp xanthum gum
- ★ 1 tsp baking powder
- ★ 25g olive oil
- ★ 75g apple juice
- ★ 1 egg

1 Preheat the oven to 180°C/gas mark 4.

2 Blanch the walnuts in boiling water for a few minutes. Drain and then chop so some of the walnuts are chunky and some are fine.

3 Mix together the flours, walnuts, xanthum gum and baking powder in a bowl.

4 In a separate bowl, whisk the olive oil, apple juice and egg until you see bubbles in the mixture.

5 Add the liquid to the flour mixture and blend into a dough. Roll out on a floured board or put a few drops of olive oil on your hands and knead the bread into the shape you want.

6 Put the loaf on a baking tray and bake for about 40 minutes until golden brown and sounding hollow when you tap the bottom.

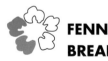

FENNEL BREAD

A chewy, rustic loaf – to make it sweeter, substitute 50ml pear juice for 50ml of the goat's milk.

MAKES 1 MEDIUM LOAF

- ★ 110g spelt flour
- ★ 60g buckwheat flour
- ★ 1 tsp baking powder
- ★ 1 tsp xanthum gum
- ★ 100ml goat's milk
- ★ 50ml goat's yoghurt
- ★ 1 egg
- ★ ½ fennel bulb, finely chopped
- ★ 1 tbsp finely chopped fennel tops (optional)

1 Preheat the oven to 180°C/gas mark 4.

2 Mix the flours, baking powder and xanthum gum in a bowl.

3 In a separate bowl, blend the milk, yoghurt and egg for 1 minute until bubbling.

4 Add the fennel bulb to the flour mixture. Make a well and stir in the milk mixture until the dough is thick and handling well. (To give the bread extra flavour, you can add the fennel tops now, if using.)

5 Shape the dough into a loaf, place on a baking tray and bake for 35–40 minutes until golden brown and sounding hollow when you tap the bottom.

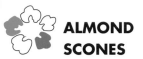 ## ALMOND SCONES

These nutty, fruity scones can be eaten hot or cold, or cut in half and toasted. Delicious with goat's butter and sugar-free jam, they will keep for 2 days, although are best eaten the day they are made.

MAKES 6

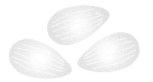

★ 75g raisins
★ 220g kamut flour
★ 1 tsp baking powder
★ 1 tsp xanthum gum
★ 110g goat's butter, softened
★ 2 tsp almond paste (see page 147) or crushed almonds
★ 1 egg
★ 70ml Almond Milk (see page 147)

1 Preheat the oven to 220°C/gas mark 7.

2 Pour enough boiling water over the raisins to cover them and leave them to soak for a few minutes. Then drain and mix in a bowl with the flour, baking powder and xanthum gum.

3 In a separate bowl, mix the softened butter and almond paste together.

4 Beat the egg and slowly mix it with the butter. Stir in the Almond Milk.

5 Make a well in the dry mix and slowly add the liquid, stirring to make a doughy paste (you may not need all the liquid).

6 Put some flour on a work surface, then roll and flatten the dough to about 5cm thick. Cut into rounds with a small biscuit cutter.

7 Place the scones on a baking tray and bake for 15–20 minutes or until golden.

ORANGE, ALMOND & SWEET POTATO CAKE

Light and moist, with no added sugar or fat, this antioxidant-rich cake is a youthing treat. It will keep in an airtight tin for about 3 days.

MAKES 6

- ★ 150g unsulphured dried apricots
- ★ 125g sweet potatoes, peeled and chopped
- ★ 3 eggs
- ★ A few drops each of vanilla and almond extracts
- ★ Grated zest and juice of 1 orange
- ★ 90g ground almonds
- ★ 90g rice flour
- ★ 1 tsp baking powder

FOR THE HOT ORANGE SYRUP
- ★ Juice of 2 oranges

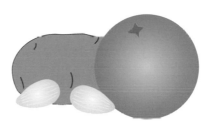

1 Preheat the oven to 180°C/gas mark 4. Grease a deep 20cm-diameter cake tin with goat's butter.

2 Pour enough boiling water over the apricots to cover them and leave to soak for 1 minute. Drain and finely chop three-quarters of them.

3 Put the sweet potatoes and chopped apricots into a saucepan with 125ml water at a low heat, and cook gently for 20–30 minutes until soft, adding more water if needed. (Most of the water should have absorbed by the end of cooking.) Take off the heat and leave to cool.

4 Separate the eggs. Put the egg whites in a clean bowl and whisk until stiff.

5 Put the sweet potato mixture, remaining apricots, vanilla and almond extracts, grated zest and orange juice, and egg yolks into a liquidizer and blend until puréed.

6 Gently fold the egg whites into the sweet potato mixture in a figure of eight. Very gently fold in the ground almonds, rice flour and baking powder.

7 Spoon the cake mixture into the prepared tin, smoothing the top with a palette knife. Bake for 30–40 minutes or until the top browns and a skewer comes out clean.

8 Meanwhile, make the hot orange syrup: pour the orange juice into a small pan, and boil until syrupy and reduced by half.

9 Turn the cake out after 10 minutes and pour the syrup over. It is delicious eaten hot or cold.

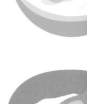
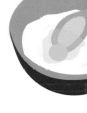
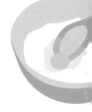
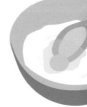
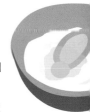
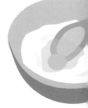

Kitchen basics

Having these basics in your larder will make cooking much easier and more flavoursome, helping you to keep eating the youthing way.

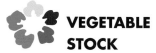 **VEGETABLE STOCK**

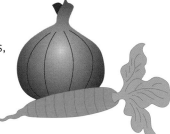

A rich, flavourful stock is the key ingredient for tasty casseroles, risottos and soups. It keeps in the fridge for 5 days or freeze in 500ml bags so you always have some handy.

MAKES ABOUT 1.5 LITRES

- ★ 2 carrots, peeled and cut lengthways
- ★ ½ head celery, roughly chopped
- ★ 2 onions, peeled and cut in halves
- ★ ¼ small turnip, peeled and chopped
- ★ 1 parsnip, peeled and cut lengthways
- ★ 1 leek, trimmed and split lengthways
- ★ 6 cabbage leaves
- ★ Small bunch parsley stalks
- ★ 4 black peppercorns
- ★ 3 bay leaves

1 Place all the ingredients in a large heavy-based pan with 6 litres water, and bring to the boil over a high heat.

2 Reduce the heat and leave to simmer for 2 hours or until reduced to about a third.

3 Strain through a colander or sieve into a clean bowl, and leave to cool.

 OVEN-DRIED TOMATOES

A fantastic way of using up extra tomatoes or those that are just going over. The best time to make this is just before you go to bed as the tomatoes can dehydrate while you are asleep. They will keep in a sealed container for up to 3 weeks in the fridge.

- ★ Tomatoes, any kind, any amount
- ★ Olive oil, to cover

1 Preheat the oven to 150°C/gas mark 2.

2 Chop the tomatoes in half, and place on a baking tray. Cook in the oven for about an hour, then switch it off and go to bed.

3 In the morning, take the tomatoes out of the oven, making sure they are completely cold. Put them in a bowl and drizzle oil over to cover them totally.

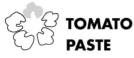 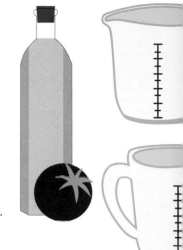

TOMATO PASTE

Use in stews, soups, pasta dishes .... Add garlic or herbs to give a richer flavour. The paste will keep in the fridge for 1 week.

MAKES ABOUT 4 TBSP

★ 4 oven-dried tomatoes (see page opposite)
★ 2 tbsp olive oil

1 Put the tomatoes and oil in a liquidizer and blend to make a paste.

QUICK TOMATO SAUCE

A quick and easy sauce for use on pasta, pizza, beans and other Italian tomato-type dishes. It will keep for 1 week in the fridge.

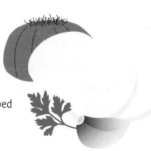

SERVES 4

★ ½ tsp coconut oil
★ ½ onion, peeled and roughly chopped
★ 2 garlic cloves, peeled and finely chopped
★ 8 tomatoes, peeled (see page 101) and roughly chopped
★ 1 tbsp finely chopped basil
★ 1 tbsp finely chopped parsley
★ 1 tbsp Tomato Paste (see above)

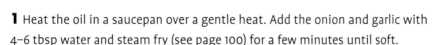

1 Heat the oil in a saucepan over a gentle heat. Add the onion and garlic with 4–6 tbsp water and steam fry (see page 100) for a few minutes until soft.
2 Add the tomatoes, and continue to cook, stirring in a little water as needed if the mixture is too dry. Keep cooking and stirring from time to time until the tomatoes break down.
3 At the last minute when the tomatoes have broken down, stir in the herbs and Tomato Paste. Using a hand-held mixer or liquidizer, blend to make a smooth tomato sauce.

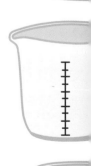

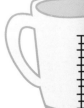

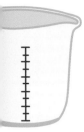

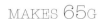 **GREEN
THAI PASTE**

Easy to make, fresh-tasting and highly youthing, this paste is the foundation of many Thai dishes. Use it in soups, curries, on salads and in salad dressings. It will keep in the fridge for 1 week.

MAKES 65G

- ★ 2 sticks lemongrass
- ★ 3 garlic cloves, peeled and finely chopped
- ★ 2cm fresh root ginger, peeled and finely chopped
- ★ ½ medium-hot red or green chilli, de-seeded and finely chopped
- ★ 1 tbsp finely chopped mint
- ★ 1 tbsp finely chopped coriander
- ★ 5 kaffir lime leaves, stalks removed and leaves chopped
- ★ 3 dry slices galangal, peeled and finely chopped
- ★ 2 spring onions, trimmed and finely chopped
- ★ 3 tbsp coconut milk (optional)

1 Remove the outer leaves from the lemongrass and cut off the thin ends. Bash the remaining stalk with the back of the knife, then chop finely.
2 Put in a large bowl with all the other ingredients and mix together to make a paste. To make a smoother paste, blend in a liquidizer with the coconut milk.

 **'CHEESE'
SPRINKLE**

A dairy-free 'cheese', use this to sprinkle on salads, pasta and rice dishes as you would Parmesan. Store in a covered pot – it will keep in the fridge for up to 2 weeks.

MAKES ABOUT 55G

- ★ 55g walnuts
- ★ 3 tbsp nutritional yeast
- ★ Large pinch mineral salt

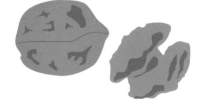

1 Put all the ingredients into a food processor and whiz until finely chopped.

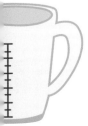

ALMOND/CASHEW BUTTER

Make this protein and antioxidant-rich nut butter as smooth or crunchy as you like. It is delicious with breads, crackers and raw veg and will last for 1 week.

MAKES 1 POT

* ★ 100g whole almonds (peeled is fine)/cashew nuts OR
  50g pumpkin seeds and 50g almonds/cashew nuts
* ★ 3 tbsp unfiltered cold-pressed extra-virgin olive oil

1 Pour enough boiling water over the almonds or cashew nuts to cover them and leave for a few minutes. Drain and then put the nuts into a liquidizer or food processor and whiz until you get the texture and consistency you're after – the longer you whiz, the smoother.
2 Stir in the oil. If the butter seems a little dry, stir in a little more oil. Place in a glass jam jar with a screw-top lid.
3 Store in the fridge and stir before using.

 ## SWEET APRICOT PASTE

This is my number one sugar substitute – use it instead of jam on toast, and in puddings and yoghurts. Store in a glass jar in the fridge, for up to 3 weeks.

MAKES 1 POT (225G)

* ★ 110g dried unsulphured apricots (or stoned dates)
* ★ 150ml freshly squeezed orange juice
* ★ 2–4 tbsp ground hemp, flax, pumpkin or sunflower seeds (optional)

1 Pour enough boiling water over the apricots (or dates if using) to cover them and leave to soak for 1 minute. Drain and then put the apricots in a bowl with the orange juice and 150ml water and leave to soak for 2–3 hours until they are swollen and plumped up.
2 Blend the apricots, juice and ground seeds (if using) in a liquidizer or food processor to a smooth paste.

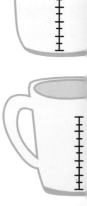

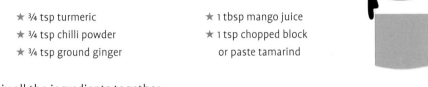

✿ YOUTHING TURMERIC PASTE

Steam frying fish, chicken or veg in this paste gives extra flavour to make a quick, simple supper dish.

MAKES 1 BATCH

- ★ ¾ tsp turmeric
- ★ ¾ tsp chilli powder
- ★ ¾ tsp ground ginger
- ★ 1 tbsp mango juice
- ★ 1 tsp chopped block or paste tamarind

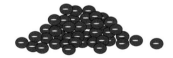

1 Mix all the ingredients together.

2 Heat a frying pan and steam fry (see page 100) fish, chicken or vegetables in the paste to give them a deep, rich taste.

3 Add water to cook thoroughly until the fish/chicken/veg is soft and the liquid has reduced by about half. Serve with rice or another grain.

✿ SWEET ADUKI BEAN PASTE

A classic Japanese paste used as a filling for cakes, pancakes or to jazz up a sweet dish – or put in a jar for use any time.

MAKES 1 SMALL POT

- ★ 200g dried aduki beans
- ★ 200g Sweet Apricot Paste (see page 145)

1 Put the beans in a large heavy-based pan and pour over enough water to cover them. Bring to the boil and drain to get rid of the toxins.

2 Return the drained beans to the pan, add 750ml water and leave the beans to soak for about 24 hours. Discard any beans that float on the top.

3 Bring the beans and soaking water to a rolling boil, then reduce the heat and simmer for about 1 hour. Add water from time to time to prevent the beans from drying out and stir frequently with a wooden spoon until the beans are very soft and the water is almost absorbed.

4 Add the Sweet Apricot (or date) Paste. Keep stirring until the beans are all crushed into a paste. Allow to cool.

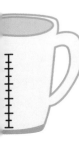
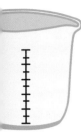

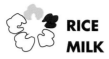 ## RICE MILK

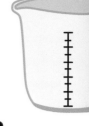

Use as milk, and in recipes as a thickener or replacement for cream. To make it sweeter, add a little grape juice or some liquidized dates. Store the milk in the fridge where it will keep for 3–4 days.

MAKES 400ML

* ★ 1 vanilla pod
* ★ 60g brown rice

1 Slice the vanilla pod down the middle. Run the tip of the knife inside the pod to scoop out all the seeds. Discard the pod.

2 In a pan, put the rice and vanilla seeds, add 600ml water and boil until the rice is very soft. Allow to cool – this will take about 1 hour in total.

3 When cool, strain through muslin or a sieve and store the milk in a jug. Eat or discard the rice.

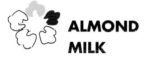 ## ALMOND MILK

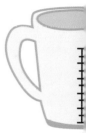

Creamy and nutritious, nut milks can be used instead of cow's milk on cereals, porridge, in hot chocolate (sweeten with grape juice or liquidized dates) or as a refreshing drink. Try cashew nut milk too. Store the milk in the fridge where it will keep for 3–4 days.

MAKES ABOUT 450ML

* ★ 140g almonds/cashew nuts (skins off)

1 Soak the almonds in enough boiling water to cover them for a few minutes. Drain and then put the almonds in a bowl and cover with a generous amount of water to allow them to expand. Leave to soak for a few hours or overnight.

2 Drain the almonds again and put them, together with 480ml fresh water, in a liquidizer. Whiz until completely smooth.

3 Strain through muslin or a sieve and store the milk in a jar. The leftover almond paste can be potted and used later in cakes and breads.

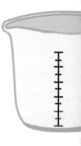

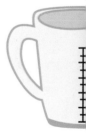

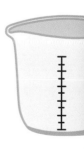

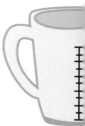

7

SUSTAINING YOUTHING FOR LIFE

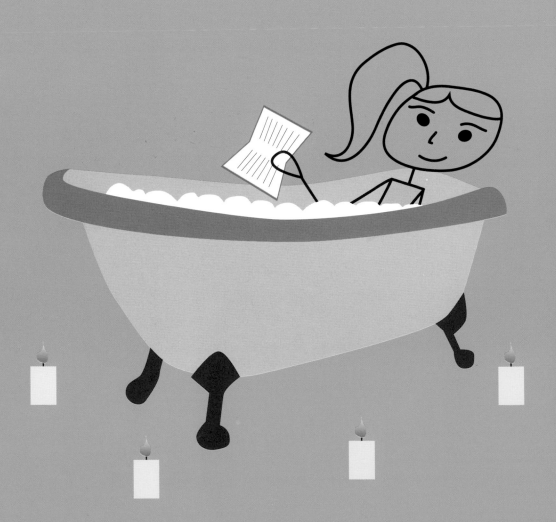

Small changes to your routine and attitudes around food, cooking and health can **re-awaken a more energetic outlook on life** to help you eat, feel and live younger. In this chapter, you'll find ways to establish youthing changes at work and home; advice on how to get those around you on board; and practical hints for eating youthfully while travelling and on holiday.

Youthing is not just about becoming less wrinkly. It is about **empowerment, energy, verve, adaptability** and the drive to truly sustain vibrancy and enjoy being the best you can be. Change always involves challenge, both mental and physical, and it tends to come when you are least expecting it. So I've also included simple tips on how to **reframe your mindset and minimize temptation,** so youthing becomes second nature not a battle against the odds. Read on: my hope is that these pages will help you avoid the tempting parking spaces on the road to success, and sustain a youthing eating programme that will **nourish you for life.**

'The road to success is dotted with many tempting parking places'

ANON

Sustainable youthing

Here are some simple rules to help you build a more youth-enhancing attitude to food and life.

ESTABLISH A ROUTINE

Eat your meals at around the same time every day. This is hugely important, because it relieves the body's anxiety around food, as well as regulating blood sugar and metabolism.

People who eat regularly have smaller waist sizes, fewer blood lipid disorders and are less likely to develop insulin resistance.

Sometimes setting regular mealtimes can meet resistance from partners, family and housemates. Children are easy as they need regular feeding, but if other people can't or won't slot in with a set time for dinner, be firm – if necessary, eat by yourself at your regular time. By following the **EYY Eating Plan** you are doing something important for yourself, and you need to be a little bit selfish. If you are always compromizing, you won't achieve the best results. If the family do complain, then make a big pot of say, coconut dhal, divide it into single portions, freeze and bring it out for yourself when you don't want to eat the family meal.

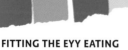

FITTING THE EYY EATING PLAN INTO FAMILY LIFE
TRY NOT TO MAKE A BIG DEAL OF IT. THE **EYY EATING PLAN** IS HEALTHY AND ENERGIZING WHATEVER YOUR AGE AND EVERYONE WILL GREATLY BENEFIT FROM AVOIDING SUGARY AND PROCESSED FOODS. SO JUST DISH IT UP AND SEE WHAT THEY SAY. IF THEY NEED TO ADD SALT, MAKE SURE IT IS MINERAL SALT, OR USE HONEY FOR SWEETNESS – AND THIS CAN BE DONE AT THE TABLE.

DON'T SKIP MEALS

When you get very hungry after missing a meal, research shows your brain craves high-fat, high-carb foods like doughnuts over more youthing choices like veg, wholegrains or fruit. So you're more likely **to pig out on fattening, anti-youthing junk food.** Brain scans show that this is an unconscious process – willpower has nothing to do with it. You can't control this brain impulse, but you can minimize its impact by *not skipping meals*.

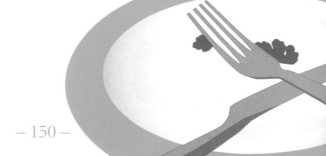

– 150 –

DRINK YOUR FOOD AND EAT YOUR JUICE

That sounds counterintuitive, but it's the most youthing way to eat. *Chew your food* until it becomes almost liquid (following the 20 second/40 second rule in the **EYY Detox** chapter, see page 78). *Always drink juice very slowly,* sipping small mouthfuls and running it around your mouth before swallowing, to give your stomach enzymes time to kick into action.

IF YOU ARE AN OVEREATER: PLATE YOUR FOOD

Plate your food, every meal, every day (see page 89). Don't have second helpings, and don't bolt food – if you're eating a meal in less than 20 minutes, you need to slow down. Download the Eat to the Beat chewing app from www.epjhealth.com to help. It's also important for you to be conscious and mindful about *not picking between meals.* That way your body gets used to being fed only at mealtimes, which will regulate appetite and make it easier to control impulsive over-eating behaviour.

IF YOU ARE AN UNDEREATER: EAT EVERYTHING ON YOUR PLATE

If you're an undereater, you need discipline around food just as much as an overeater. You need to plate yourself, and eat everything on your plate – with no excuses. For the first week, ask someone else to plate food for you, so you have no choice but to eat a set amount. At least twice a week after a meal, have a pudding. Don't pick between meals, as that can give you an excuse not to eat the next meal. It's important for you to have very regular mealtimes – within a 15-minute time frame every day (for example, eat breakfast at 7–7.15am; lunch at 12.45–1pm; dinner at 6.30–6.45pm). When you've been undereating, your body goes into shutdown and stores fat to protect itself, and you start to think about food all the time. But when you feed your body regularly, cravings stop, metabolism regulates and *you spend much less time obsessing about food.* Eating becomes like brushing your teeth – something you do without thinking too much about it.

EAT UP?

In Russia and China, it's rude not to leave a bit of food on a plate (to show you're satisfied and have had your fill); whereas in Japan and Britain, leaving food can indicate you didn't like the meal. Some people have to eat everything on their plate, no matter how full they are – throwing away food is a big no-no drummed into them in childhood. Try and free yourself from these mindsets: eat until you are about two-thirds full (unless you are an over- or undereater, in which case see page 151).

RETHINK YOUR TREATS

If bad moods have an impact on what you eat – for example, you scoff comfort foods when something upsets you – then redesign your concept of a treat. Instead of thinking chips, burgers, ice cream, chocolate or alcohol, go for something high in fibre like mashed potatoes, porridge, a fruit crumble or a bowl of banana, dates and sheep's yoghurt (or any other **EYY** pudding). It'll satisfy you and have *youthing benefits* too. Or, better still, think about treats as pampering yourself with a long, lush bath or dancing naked to your favourite tunes. Whatever moves you in a positive way.

> *Don't bother keeping a food diary. You'd think it would help to monitor your food intake, but research shows people forget to write down all the foods they eat, and underestimate amounts hugely. It's better to regulate intake by plating food and eating three meals a day.*

STICK WITH IT

Many of my clients feel desperate when they 'fall off' the **EYY Eating Plan** and pig out on something they think they shouldn't. But I always say, *don't beat yourself up,* it really doesn't matter. This way of eating is for life and having one junk meal or too much wine is not going to negate the rest of your youthing work. It's better to think of the **EYY Eating Plan** as a journey and look for ways in which you're progressing, rather than focusing on how you are falling short.

Take the opportunity to reassess your aims: look back at Chapter 4, *evaluate the progress you've made,* and reassess the youthing goals you still hope to reach. It also might be worth building a wider variety of foods into your diet: sometimes a craving can be an indication that not all your nutritional needs are being met.

Eating out

You can eat out the **EYY** way at most restaurants and cafés. It's usually fairly easy to make good youthing choices from the menu: think grilled, steamed or poached meat and fish; raw or steamed veg; light soups, dips like guacamole, salsa or hummus, grilled goat's cheese for starters. Fill up on a salad first and eat a sensible ratio of heathy foods: for example, two courses of youthing foods to one non-youthing. Choose wholemeal pasta and brown rice, ask the kitchen to hold the sugar, salt and soy, and ask for salad dressings to be served on the side. If there's nothing suitable on the menu, ask the chef to make you something simple like an omelette.

DINNER WITH FRIENDS

It can be difficult to eat youthing foods when you're at someone's house for dinner (self-serve buffets are much easier!). Most hosts nowadays ask for their guests' food preferences beforehand – tell them that you're on a special diet eating lots of veg, fruit and fish and steering clear of sugar and meat. Say it sounds difficult but you are happy to bring along your own main dish, rather than have them make something special for you – you can eat their salad or veg sides along with it. Fresh fruit puddings are easy to organize.

　　Things get more complicated when you are meeting someone for the first time and want to impress them – for example, your boyfriend/girlfriend's parents. Then, I'd advise not making a big deal about your youthing preferences. **Eat a small meal before you go,** and as much of the foods as you can while you're there. They'll probably think you are nervous rather than picky. If it goes well, you can always reveal your preferences later.

YOUTHING DINNER PARTY

You want to host a dinner party but are worried that people won't like eating foods with no sugar, salt or bad fats? No problem: try them on the menu overleaf – so delicious, flavoursome and satisfying, they won't notice a thing.

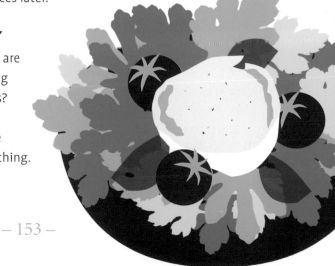

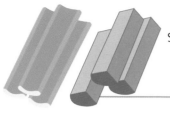

PRE-DINNER NIBBLES

Spicy Chickpeas (see page 136) and raw crudités **with**
Avocado Summer Dip (see page 137) **and**
Super Youthing Salsa (see page 136)

STARTER

Youthing Butternut Squash and Ginger Soup (see
page 114) **with** Walnut Bread (see page 139)

MAIN

Cod with Mango (see page 118) **or**
Spinach-stuffed Salmon (see page 122) on a bed of mandolined courgettes **with**
Garlic and Ginger Broccoli (see page 127)
Antioxidant Aubergines (see page 124)

PUDDING

Youthing Summer Pudding (see page 134) **or**
Detox Apple Tart (see page 135) **with**
Vanilla Soya Custard (see page 133)

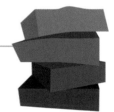

FOR AFTERS

Tiny cubes of Beanie Brownie (see page 133) to serve
as petit-fours with after-dinner coffee/tea.

ON HOLIDAY

If you're staying in a hotel, phone or email
ahead of your arrival and tell them your dietary
requirements – hotels are used to dealing with
many different requests and eating regimes.

★ Before you go, learn a few standard phrases in
the native language – for example, 'Please can
I have steamed veg' or 'Can you make this
without salt/sugar?'

★ Take your favourite foods with you: sprouted
breads, liquid aminos, seeds and nuts, salad dressings – whatever you
think you might not be able to find abroad. Don't worry about fresh fruit
and veg – these are almost always available.

> When you're
> cooking or making a big
> salad for everyone, take out a
> portion for yourself before adding
> the final cream, cheese or dressing –
> that way, everyone gets to eat
> the way they want.

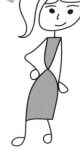

★ If you're staying in a self-catering villa/apartment with friends, 'fess up before you go. Instead of being shy and getting bullied into eating things you don't want, learn to laugh at yourself. I always say: 'I know, I am the most impossible person in the world, I can't help it, I just love the food I love – I'll make my own so nobody else has to worry about it.' Half the time people become so curious they end up eating what I'm having anyway and rather enjoy it. But if not, then it's a way of your differences being in the open so you won't feel guilty or embarrassed that you're inconveniencing everyone else, and can eat as you want.

GETTING THERE

On trains and planes, I always take some nibbles with me: a big bag of raw veg or carrot and pepper sticks, nuts, seeds, raisins or other dried fruit, oatcakes, my own breads, hard-boiled eggs, sliced goat's cheese, even a baked potato or some rice cooked with veg and olive oil to eat cold. It means you can have a meal without eating highly processed plane food.

> *Don't buy pre-prepared vegetables and fruits from supermarkets or cafés – they often have additives to keep them looking fresh, and as soon as they are cut (probably several days ago), they start to lose their nutritional value.*

AT THE OFFICE

It's a good idea to have plenty of youthing food choices around at work so you don't find yourself eating foods you'd rather avoid.

★ Take in lunch: many of the recipes on pages 111–16 make good lunch choices – make double the amount and save half for next day's lunch. If your workplace doesn't have facilities for heating up food, take in a flask of soup or a salad and some homemade bread.

★ If you're buying a take-away lunch, choose youthing options: a baked potato, salad, soup. Some cafés and high street food chains provide healthier, fresher foods than others – research the ones closest to your workplace.

★ Keep basics like olive oil and lemon at work for drizzling over salads and baked potatoes.

★ Always have snacks in your desk drawer, such as seeds, nuts, chopped vegetables and fresh fruit, to stave off hunger in case you can't leave the office on time.

Be your biggest supporter

A bit of body maintenance can go a long way towards helping you feel more relaxed and in tune with your aims and emotions.

Body scrub: give yourself an occasional mineral salt scrub in the shower, rinsing well all over afterwards. It stimulates circulation, helping with detox and alkalization.

Tongue scraping: removing bacteria, fungi and food debris from the tongue removes over 80% of the oral bacteria that cause bad breath and are linked with ageing health problems such as heart disease. Use a specially designed tongue scraper or small metal spoon. Scrape your tongue from the back to the front first thing in the morning before eating or drinking anything. The debris may be thick, white, brown or yellow. After a while on the **EYY Detox** and **EYY Eating Plan**, you'll notice the coating on your tongue will change to become a thin white film – this is a sign that your body is healthy and *in the optimum state for youthing.*

Make your own body scrub with a handful of mint, rosemary and lavender mixed with half a cup of sea salt, saturated with olive oil. Alternatively, rub coffee grounds from a cafetière on your skin in the shower.

Take exercise: good muscle tone is youthing, and exercise has an afterburn effect – your metabolism is higher for 24 hours afterwards. Exercise gives you a lean physique, helps balance hormones, creates stamina and *raises your emotional and mental energy* – all highly youthing. Even jiggling around a lot, taking the stairs instead of the lift, stretching or jogging on the spot while you're making a cup of tea, burns extra energy each day. Push yourself to achieve more physically each week and you'll not only feel more youthful but will be less likely to give in to cravings and comfort food messages from the brain.

See also the herbal helpers on page 81.

BRAIN TRAINING

The way we eat is often linked to the way we think about food. Here are some tips for silencing your inner saboteur.

1 **Control the backchat:** if you walk past a sweet shop every day and your brain starts obsessing about a chocolate bar in the window, you know you're self-sabotaging. Recognize the signs, then rein in the backchat by asking: am I hungry, and is this the food that will be most youthing to eat? Walk on by, and most times you will have forgotten the chocolate in 10 minutes.

2 **Define temptation:** temptation is not about what food is on offer around you, but about what is going on in your head. Realize that you grow stronger by sticking to your beliefs and aims around food, and weaker and less confident every time you undermine them.

3 **Don't limit yourself** by setting 'achievable' goals at the start. Instead, wait to see how you look and feel after detox and a few weeks on the **EYY Eating Plan** – your confidence will grow, possibilities will open up and the world will seem a more exciting place. Then is the time to set any future youthing goals.

4 **Rethink yourself:** if you are someone who traditionally beats yourself up over the smallest thing, has been on 100 diets and considers yourself a failure because none have worked; then don't do that to yourself. This is not what **EYY** is about. It's not a punishment: it is about enjoying yourself, about reaching your potential – at heart, it's about respecting yourself, being willing to change things that have become routine and are running you rather than you running them.

5 **Feel the power:** it is a very powerful feeling when finally you do something that is just for you and no one else. You may think the only benefit of this diet and lifestyle change is to you – but is it? If your efforts reap results, your close family and friends and also wider family, workmates and acquaintances will change too. This may seem a small selfish step, but who knows where it could go. You can influence a whole generation. Revolutions start on less ...

> This is a chance to rethink your aims, rethink yourself. Remember the saying: 'The person who says it cannot be done should not interrupt the person doing it.'

Recipe index

A

aduki beans:
  beanie brownie 133
  sweet aduki bean paste 146
  vitality black bean curry 119
almonds:
  almond butter 145
  almond milk 147
  almond scones 140
  orange, almond and sweet potato cake 141
  youthing nut bars 137
apples:
  apple and carrot detox speeder 105
  detox apple tart 135
  muesli baked apples 110
  pear, apple and blueberry compote 110
apricots:
  orange, almond and sweet potato cake 141
  sweet apricot paste 145
  youthing nut bars 137
artichokes:
  energizing fennel and artichoke salad 115
Asian crunchy stir-fry 130
aubergines:
  antioxidant aubergines 124
  goat's cheese, aubergine and butter bean bake 118
avocados:
  avocado summer dip 137
  cod with mango 118
  creamy avocado dream 105

B

bananas:
  blueberry layered coulis 132

barley:
  mushroom barley risotto 126
  Thai curry with 120
beans, baked 108
beansprouts:
  Asian crunchy stir-fry 130
  super soba noodle salad 116
beetroot:
  creamy beetroot detox soup 112
  detox root and beetroot burst 104
  super-charged spring cleaner 106
  sweet beetroot slaw 114
  watercress, beetroot and carrot zinger 104
blueberries:
  blueberry layered coulis 132
  pear, apple and blueberry compote 110
  youthing summer pudding 134
borlotti bean and cavolo nero casserole 125
bread:
  pumpkin seed and tomato 138
  walnut 139
broccoli, garlic and ginger 127
buckwheat pancakes with pear, apple and blueberry compote 110
butter beans:
  goat's cheese, aubergine and butter bean bake 118
butternut squash:
  super youthing stroganoff 122
  youthing butternut squash and ginger soup 114
  youthing coconut curry 123

C

cake, orange, almond and sweet potato 141

cannellini beans:
  alkalizing cannellini bean soup 113
  baked beans 108
carrots:
  apple and carrot detox speeder 105
  go skin glow 104
  watercress, beetroot and carrot zinger 104
cashew nuts:
  cashew butter 145
  youth-boost burger 117
casserole, borlotti bean and cavolo nero 125
cauliflower:
  youthing coconut curry 123
cavolo nero and borlotti bean casserole 125
celeriac:
  super youthing stroganoff 122
'cheese' sprinkle 144
chickpeas, spicy 136
chocolate: beanie brownie 133
coconut milk:
  creamy coconut and pineapple black rice pud 131
  youthing coconut curry 123
cod with mango 118
courgettes, stuffed 128
cucumber:
  green gazpacho 111
curries:
  Thai curry with barley 120
  vitality black bean curry 119
  youthing coconut curry 123
custard, vanilla soya 133

D

dates: beanie brownie 133
dhal, soothing coconut 128–9
dip, avocado summer 137

F

fennel:
  fennel and artichoke salad
    115
  fennel bread 139–40
  fennel soup 112
figs:
  figgy nut bircher muesli 109
  pear and fig winter
    smoothie 106
fruity jelly 132

G

garlic and ginger broccoli 127
gazpacho, green 111
ginger:
  garlic and ginger broccoli
    127
goat's cheese, aubergine and
  butter bean bake 118
golden chai 107

J

jellies, fruity 132
juices 102–7

K

kidney beans:
  spiced-up beanie salad 116
  super youthing stroganoff
    122
  youth-boost burger 117

L

lentil detoxer 129
lettuce: green gazpacho 111

M

mangoes:
  cod with 118
milk:
  almond 147
  rice 147
muesli:
  homemade muesli base 109
  muesli baked apples 110

mushroom barley risotto
  126

N

nuts:
  nut butters 145
  vanilla nut shake 107
  youthing nut bars 137
  see also almonds; cashew
    nuts; walnuts

O

oats:
  figgy nut bircher muesli
    109
  homemade muesli base
    109
  youthing nut bars 137
orange, almond and sweet
  potato cake 141

P

pak choi:
  Asian crunchy stir-fry 130
pears:
  pear and fig winter
    smoothie 106
  pear, apple and blueberry
    compote 110
pineapples:
  creamy coconut and
    pineapple black rice
    pud 131
potatoes:
  antioxidant-rich potato
    salad 115
  baked potato with wasabi
    124 5
  potato juice 105
puddings 131–5

R

raspberries:
  youthing summer pudding
    134
relish, sweet tomato 117

rice:
  creamy coconut and
    pineapple black rice
    pud 131
  mushroom barley risotto 126
  rice milk 147

S

salads:
  antioxidant-rich potato 115
  energizing fennel and
    artichoke 115
  spiced-up beanie 116
  super soba noodle 116
  sweet beetroot slaw 114
salmon:
  salmon nabemono 121
  spinach-stuffed 122–3
salsa, super youthing 136
scones, almond 140
seeds:
  homemade muesli base 109
  pumpkin seed and tomato
    bread 138
  youthing nut bars 137
side dishes 127–30
snacks 136–7
soba noodle salad 116
soups:
  alkalizing cannellini bean 113
  creamy beetroot detox 112
  fennel 112
  green gazpacho 111
  youthing butternut squash
    and ginger 114
soya beans:
  super soba noodle salad 116
soya milk:
  vanilla soya custard 133
spinach:
  spinach-stuffed salmon
    122–3
  super youthing salsa 136
split peas:
  soothing coconut dhal
    128–9

stock, vegetable 142
strawberries:
    youthing summer pudding
        134
sweet potatoes:
    orange, almond and sweet
        potato cake 141

T
tart, detox apple 135
Thai curry with barley 120
Thai paste, green 144
tomatoes:
    baked beans 108
    oven-dried 142
    peppy Virgin Mary 106
    pumpkin seed and tomato
        bread 138
    quick tomato sauce 143
    sweet tomato relish 117
    tomato paste 143
    vitality black bean curry 119
turmeric paste 146

V
vanilla:
    vanilla nut shake 107
    vanilla soya custard 133
vegetables:
    detox root and beetroot
        burst 104
    roasted root vegetables 127
    vegetable stock 142
W
walnuts:
    'cheese' sprinkle 144
    figgy nut bircher muesli 109
    spinach-stuffed salmon
        122–3
    walnut bread 139
watercress, beetroot and
    carrot zinger 104
Y
yoghurt:
    blueberry layered coulis 132

Acknowledgements

I would like to dedicate this book to my Aunt Peggy who since the beginning of my journey has consistently been there to pick me up and guide me, listen to me, wipe my brow, encourage me and hold my hand. She is the embodiment of youthful energy, who remains ageless, elegant and fascinating. She is my inspiration.

I'd also like to thank my husband, mother and sisters who have been incredibly long-suffering with my moans and unavailability. My agent Heather Holden Brown, who took me on and had faith even when I had given up, and Anne Furniss of Quadrille who, in the early days, saw something worth backing and has been wonderfully supportive throughout. Everyone will thank Jane Phillimore who has made this script readable and more importantly fun!

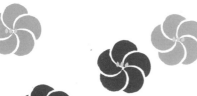